CHASING CUPCAKES

Chasing Cupcakes

How One Broke, Fat Girl Transformed
Her Life (and How You Can, Too)

E L I Z A B E T H   B E N T O N

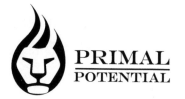

CHASING CUPCAKES

How One Broke, Fat Girl Transformed
Her Life (and How You Can, Too)

ISBN   978-1-5445-0127-7   *Hardcover*

        978-1-5445-0124-6   *Paperback*

        978-1-5445-0125-3   *Ebook*

        978-1-5445-0126-0   *Audiobook*

*To Betsy and to everyone out there who feels like she did—
exhausted by the struggle to create change and find happiness,
but unwilling to let go of the hope that it's possible. To all those
who refuse to give up. To the tired fighters who believe in the
veracity of their potential. To those who doubt themselves, who
feel perpetually in their own way and desperately want to change
their lives: it **is** possible for you. It can be easier. It **will be** easier.*

*As we navigate these pages and you transition into effective, life-
enhancing action, I am here with you and for you. I'm here to
help you thrive through this transformation, not simply survive
it. **Your journey is where the joy is** and I'm here to help you
come alive. Change is right over the horizon. It's much closer
than you think. Let's go there together, one choice at a time.*

Contents

*"When I let go of what I am,
I become what I might be."*

—LAO TZU

Prologue

"It's okay. It's...okay." There was something about her reserved tone, like she was trying to convince herself or maybe to swallow the sound of shame. There was an obvious sadness in her voice and on her face.

She was my mom, standing next to me in the only full bathroom in our colonial New England home. I was seven years old, wearing only my underwear, standing on the bathroom scale, embarrassed.

"It's okay," she said again, to both of us. "You just tell yourself that this is the heaviest day of your life." She emphasized those last words, **heaviest day of your life**, as if they were an unwavering declaration. She wanted me to remember them, believe them, and commit to them.

For the first time, the scale below me was displaying *triple digits*. I weighed one hundred pounds.

The heaviest day of my life, she'd said. Looking back, I can muster a weak laugh at the irony. It was the *lightest* I'd ever be.

But I wasn't laughing then. It was awkward for both of us. I remember feeling huge, like I was taking up all the space in the room. But at the same time, I felt so small. Ashamed. I wanted to disappear—a feeling I'd grow very accustomed to over the next couple decades.

I burst into tears.

My weight had been creeping up. Maybe soaring up...I don't remember. That was the reason my mom created the new rule: I had to check my weight in front of her every morning.

Her expectation was unspoken but clear: my weight could only go down from this point forward. She was going to do **everything** in her power to make sure it did.

Though the weigh-ins only lasted a few minutes of each day, they consumed my mind all day and night. I'd go to bed anxious and wake up desperate to do whatever possible to weigh even the slightest bit less than the day before. I'd frantically and repeatedly spit into a cup. I'd cut my own hair. I'd turn the shower on so the bathroom would fill with steam and quietly do jumping jacks, believing I could sweat out a half pound in the three minutes before my mom walked in. Anything at all to make the scale display a number that wouldn't disappoint my mom and embarrass me.

Looking back, my approach was irrational and emotional. I was in a frantic pursuit to simply drive down the number on the scale. I was waging a battle against the scale; fighting against my body instead of working with it. I wanted acceptance from my mom and my peers, and I felt the only way to be accepted (and acceptable) was to lose weight.

Unfortunately, I didn't get that acceptance and I didn't escape embarrassment. In fact, rejection and shame followed me everywhere I went. My weight kept climbing. The bigger I got, the smaller and less significant I felt.

Shortly after the daily weigh-in was instituted, my mom layered on a second element to my unwelcome morning routine: running. She'd wake me up early to run two miles before school. I always complained and made excuses, but she didn't waver. She embodied a motivation and commitment I lacked.

We lived on Main Street, appropriately the primary road

in our small New Hampshire town. I was young and my mom wanted me to be safe, so she bought me an orange traffic vest—you know, one of the reflective ones—and would often follow me in the car.

I hated running. It felt like a punishment. I was tired and wanted to be in bed, like my sister who was still asleep at home. Instead, I was out running, dressed to draw attention, every passerby unable to ignore the neon fat kid shuffling down the road, wood-paneled Pontiac station wagon crawling eerily behind.

On busy mornings, my mom wouldn't have time to follow in the car. I *loved* those days. When she wasn't watching, I would jog just to the nearby church parking lot and hide in the back, sitting against the trees so she wouldn't see me if she came looking. This was before cell phones, so I had no way to entertain myself. I'd just sit and feel sorry for myself, waiting for the time to pass. I'd wish I wasn't so different, wasn't so fat. Or, I'd wish I had something to eat. At an early age, food had already become both escape and rebellion.

At one point, my mom paid my sister Debi, two years older, to be my "trainer." In fact, this was Debi's "job" for a couple summers: underage personal trainer to her fat sister. I vividly remember the orange plastic whistle she'd blow as I ran sprints up and down the driveway.

Debi was a natural athlete. She was built like a gazelle: much taller than I was, with long, lean legs and not an ounce of extra fat on her. I, on the other hand, was built like a dump truck with four flat tires carrying an oversize load. No one ever commented on our resemblance. You're shocked, I'm sure.

Debi ran cross-country in middle school, so for scheduling ease and as a way to ensure I was exercising enough to offset my weight problem, my mom insisted I join the team as well. Clearly, there weren't tryouts. I was *awful*. While Debi came in first in every race and every practice, I came in last.

When I say that I came in last, I don't mean I was trailing toward the back of the pack. I was so far *behind* the pack, I couldn't see my teammates. I probably didn't even know there *was* a pack—that the rest of the kids ran *together*. I would finish so far behind everyone else that the coaches often sent kids out to look for me. I wasn't lost. I was just *really* slow.

My slowness, fatness, and routine search-and-rescue requirements during practice and meets were great fodder for insults and jokes at my expense.

In third grade, we were reading a *Magic School Bus* book about space travel. My whole class was sitting at the front of the room when a classmate turned to me and shouted, "You're so fat you sink in gravity!" Everyone laughed. Even if I had been quick enough to realize that we *all* sink in gravity (I wasn't), the point had been made. The punch had been thrown. I was fat.

I went home and told my parents what the boy had said. My dad told me to go back the next day and tell him that he's such an airhead, he floats!

I did. His response hit harder than mine, "Well, at least I'm not fat!" Fair point. In the third grade, thin was a greater prize than smart. Fat was a harsher shame than stupid.

I stopped defending myself. At home and at school, **fat seemed indefensible.**

A couple years later, when girls in my class saw me eating watermelon and swallowing the seeds, they passed a note around the table joking that I had watermelons growing in my stomach. I remember wanting to tell them that wasn't true—that swallowing the seeds didn't make watermelons grow inside you—but stopping myself because I'd rather them blame my size on fruit than fat. Fat seemed worse. I stayed quiet and let them whisper about my weight.

It was a weird feeling, getting bigger and feeling

smaller, at the same time. It was a feeling I'd try to escape from, and food became my anesthetic.

I isolated myself. I believed that being fat meant being unlikeable and I didn't know any other way to protect myself from rejection. I didn't know much, but I was *certain* I wasn't good enough. My insecurities about my weight led to me not wanting to eat in front of other people. Eating would only draw attention to my weight. I compensated by binging when I was alone. It felt like a relief to eat when no one was watching or judging. I got heavier and heavier.

Years later, I'd talk about these feelings with my mom—on my podcast, of all places, with thousands of people listening. At the start of the conversation, I explained to her that, growing up, I just had a sense that I wasn't enough.

"*You weren't,*" she responded, matter-of-factly.

Though it was decades later and I had matured, changed, and developed a growing self-confidence, it hurt to hear those words from her and receive that stinging confirmation.

It had always felt like rejection. It still did. It was everywhere, in almost every interaction in my life, not just with my mom. I'm pretty sure I carried it with me into each of my relationships.

As a freshman in high school, I had a boyfriend who was a senior. I was so excited when he invited me to his Senior Snowball semi-formal dance. As had already become a pattern, my mom and I decided I'd buy a dress that was too small so I'd be motivated to lose weight and fit into it.

As had *also* been a pattern, the day of the dance came and the dress was still too small. Quite a bit too small. It wouldn't zip. I was getting ready at my friend's house and I was beyond embarrassed. I didn't know what to do! We were leaving in thirty minutes and I had no other options.

My mom asked my friend's mom if they had any duct tape. She brought the shiny roll of super-adhesive tape into the guest room, I took my clothes off and she bound me tightly with it. I could barely breathe, never mind *move*, but we got the dress on and zipped. I was mortified at the way my back fat spilled out over the dress and my mom shrugged sympathetically, "You're in it. That's all we can do. But you don't ever have to feel this again."

It was a not-so-subtle weight loss reminder. *You created this problem.*

At the end of the night, as I ripped the industrial-strength tape off my bare belly and breasts, I could hear my mom's words echoing in my head: "You have to suffer to be beautiful."

I was suffering, but I didn't feel beautiful. I never had. I felt alone, defeated, and ashamed.

I turned to food to fill myself up. Not because I was hungry, but because I was empty.

It would be years before I understood that **food is only the solution when hunger is the problem.**

I had a full belly and an empty, lonely soul.

Since I felt so certain that my weight was a problem, I started doing what we're taught to do when we cause a problem: apologize. I apologized for my weight to everyone: friends, boyfriends, my high school volleyball coach, and prospective employers.

I would lead almost every introduction with the story about my weight, an apology for it, and a pledge to lose weight, like I owed it to them.

I apologized for my weight so many times that I began to identify *as* the apology. I wasn't a young woman; I wasn't a smart professional; I wasn't a feisty partner. **I was a living, breathing problem waiting for an overdue solution.**

My discomfort with my weight didn't contribute to a

solution. It drove me deeper into the problem. Shame and disgust weren't effective strategies for encouraging change. Hating my large body didn't make it smaller; I continued getting bigger. I ate more. I hid more. I enjoyed life less. Though I didn't realize it at the time, overeating didn't add pleasure to my life; it took it all away.

I struggled to break free from the problem of my weight because I identified with it. If overweight is who I am, how can I be someone else? I accepted it, sadly and with a lot of drama. While I wanted something different (confidence and weight loss were at the top of the list), I *couldn't* create those changes because I was so deeply attached to my identity as **the fat girl**. It was my beginning and my end. My weight was consuming and defining me.

I sank to my dangerously low expectations. I behaved in accordance with how I had defined myself.

I had zero respect for myself and that lack of respect spilled over into my relationships with others.

Silently, through the example of how I treated *myself*, I taught other people how to treat me.

Because I believed my weight made me unlovable, I convinced others that they should feel that way, too. I taught them to believe that I wasn't good enough. I rejected myself and indirectly suggested they should reject me, too. They bought into the story I told them about how I wasn't good enough because of my weight, and they began reinforcing that story with their actions, words, and expectations. It became a lonely, unhealthy, vicious cycle.

This pattern was most prominent in my romantic relationships. I guess, to be fair, it was most prominent in my romantic relationships because I didn't really *have* any platonic relationships after middle school. I didn't have the confidence to develop friendships. I assumed people wouldn't like me because I was fat, so I didn't even try.

I had a long-distance relationship during my freshman year of college. Against my family's wishes, I walked away from my Latin scholarship in Washington, DC, and transferred to school in North Carolina so we could be together.

He broke up with me two days after I unpacked in my new dorm. He told me he couldn't deal with my weight anymore. He wasn't attracted to me.

I was devastated. I returned to New England heartbroken, ashamed, and freshly motivated by gut-wrenching rejection. Once again, I wasn't striving for my own health or happiness; I wanted to meet someone else's standard—to become "good enough" for someone else. For months, I ate nothing but protein shakes and chicken broth. After reporting back to him with my weight loss, he agreed that we could get back together.

I moved *back* to North Carolina. I taught him, through my example, that my weight was a bargaining chip and he picked up that ball and ran with it.

For the next two years, everything in that relationship was based on whether I had lost weight or gained weight. When I lost weight, I was rewarded. When I gained weight or failed to lose weight, I was punished. There was dramatically more gaining than losing as I continued to work against my body instead of with it. I didn't see food as fuel; it was a numbing agent and something in my life that wouldn't reject me. It was a factor I could control when my mind and life felt so frighteningly out of control.

Though that relationship ended, my patterns with food and weight continued. I'd pledge to lose weight, thinking that it would come with a side of acceptance. I'd go on a crash diet, lose some weight, and, with a reduced sense of urgency, return to my previous patterns and habits: overeat, overindulge, isolate, apologize, restrict, repeat.

Permanent change and unconditional confidence felt

completely out of reach. As I saw it, I had tried to change and failed so many times, yet I wasn't getting better; I was getting worse.

I was in my late twenties, depressed, in debt, and working sixty-plus hours a week in a job that stressed me out beyond measure. I hadn't been to a doctor for a checkup in years because I couldn't bear to hear that I had tipped the scales over 350 pounds. I was married to a man I was hiding from because I hated myself so much that I couldn't possibly let him love me. I didn't believe I was lovable. I was certain it was impossible. If he told me I was beautiful, I was certain he was lying. I didn't want to go anywhere or do anything because I was too ashamed of my body.

It's impossible to genuinely connect with someone when you're trying to escape yourself.

To say that it was a dark time in my life would be a gross understatement.

My job took up most of my time and I complained about it incessantly. I complained about my bosses, the workload, the customers, my coworkers, the clients, the hours— there wasn't much I *didn't* complain about. I woke up every day with anxiety, nervous to check my email and see what problems were waiting in my inbox.

Around that time, I read a quote from the poet Rumi. It said:

"Why do you stay in prison when the door is so wide open?"

Whoa. It stopped me in my tracks. I wasn't in prison. My job *wasn't* a prison. I was walking into it every day, by choice. The door was wide open. I wasn't stuck. I wasn't there against my will. I was there by my deliberate, repetitive choices. I could find another job. No one forced me to drive there every day; no one forced me to go in early, stay late, or work weekends. I had options.

I had created my own unhappiness.

"Why do you stay in prison when the door is so wide open?"

There was no prison. I was free to change anything and everything.

I was free in general.

I realized I was living in a misery of my own making. I was living in shackles I had put on myself. **I was confined by walls I had built**—walls I was continuing to build, choice by choice.

Shackles of debt from my own spending.

Shackles of obesity from my own food choices.

Shackles of work stress from a job I applied for, accepted, and chose to stay at.

Shackles of depression from my own commitment to the problems instead of the solutions.

Shackles of loneliness because of my own decision to isolate myself.

How much of my life had I missed? Was I willing to continue missing it? Were the choices that were causing me to miss out worth it?

What was I chasing? Was it worth it?

I came to love Rumi's poetry. I bought a book of his work, *The Essential Rumi*, and was inspired by one of his pieces about, of all things, drunk people. In this long poem about the drunks stumbling around a tavern, he wrote, "Whoever brought me here will have to take me home."

Whoever brought me here will have to take me home. **I had brought myself to this dark place in my life and I was the only one who could bring myself someplace else.**

No one was coming to save me. My mom couldn't save

me. My husband couldn't save me. My sister couldn't save me. No diet had ever saved me and certainly wouldn't be able to now. Even if someone *wanted* to save me, I was the only one who could do the work. **Change would require my full and exclusive participation.** I chose my way into these circumstances and I would have to choose my way out of them.

I had spent years living and thinking in the problem. **I was so attached to the problem that I wasn't giving any energy or attention to the solution.** It was time to get out of the past, out of the story, out of the limitations I had placed on myself and into a new way of thinking about myself and my life.

Whoever brought me here would have to bring me home.

I had to do it, and it was possible. I didn't yet know *how*, but I believed I could make my present and future different from my past. I was capable of choices different from the ones I'd grown accustomed to making. I was capable of creating change. I was capable of making different choices, moment to moment. I didn't want to miss out on any more of my life. I didn't want to keep chasing the wrong things for the wrong reasons.

In the same poem about the drunks at the tavern, Rumi

explains that fermentation is one of the oldest symbols for human transformation.

In the process of fermentation, grapes are closed up in a dark place for a long time, after which the results can be spectacular, if they emerge at the right time. If they stay in the dark for too long, it can be disastrous.

I had closed myself off for years, stayed in a dark place, and made choices that kept me there, but if I emerged at the right time, the results could be transformative. Beautiful. Spectacular.

I wanted that. I knew I had to step into something new and out of something familiar. I knew that in order to step into my full potential, I had to step away from the limits of my past patterns.

It was the right time for me.

It was my moment. I was free to create change. To *be* change. To refuse to keep myself in prison.

Our patterns and stories, no matter how far back they go, can be surrendered and rewritten. We can walk away from them in any moment. Every choice can be change and every moment is a blank slate.

The way things have been does not have to be the way they continue to be.

I was inspired by an idea from Chinese philosopher Lao Tzu: "When I let go of what I am, I become what I might be." When I let go of the idea that I'm a fat girl who can't change, I can become something else.

When I stop chasing pleasure and acceptance, I can be whatever I choose to be.

In the past, I had been quick to jump to the second part without understanding the mandatory prerequisite of the first part. To become what I could be, I have to let go of what I've been. As the cliché goes, you can't steal second with your foot on first.

I had to let go. I had to stop arguing for the problem. I had to stop instructing myself to be that old version of myself so I could open myself up to new options. I had to be willing to not make old choices so I could get new results.

I knew the failed tactics of the past wouldn't be my present solutions. I had to stop hiding, stop trying to be small, and **stop confusing emptiness for hunger**. I had to stop chasing and choosing the shackles of food, spending, and my past so that I could set myself free.

I couldn't hate my way to self-respect. I couldn't restrict my way to a healthy relationship with food. I had to work *with* my body instead of against it.

There were a lot of things I had to unlearn to go from depressed, isolated, obese, food-obsessed, lazy, and in debt to a fit, healthy, confident, debt-free, joyful business owner.

In the coming chapters, I'll share with you how I did it, how you can do it, and how to incorporate these strategies into your full, busy life. I'll share tactics for overcoming excuses and practicing incremental yet dramatic change, no matter how strong the chains to your past and your patterns feel.

These strategies helped me pay off over $130,000 in debt. They helped me start a business that has always been and remains debt-free. These strategies helped me create confidence for the first time in my life. They helped me fall in love with fitness, despite a lifetime of resisting and resenting it. They helped me lose 150 pounds and they helped me take great care of myself, even during the most difficult periods of my life.

These strategies transformed my life in every way possible. Transformation is available to you, too, and we'll create it together.

This is the book I wish I had when I felt hopeless and overwhelmed. This is the book I wish I had to walk me through the daily process of creating change. This book will help you break free from patterns, limitations, and destructive beliefs and create a life of freedom, confidence, and achievement.

The right time is right now.

Let's get started.

Getting the Most Out of This Book

"It will generally be admitted that the true test of all books is the influence they have upon the lives and conduct of their readers."

—CHARLES HELMAN LEA

This quote perfectly captures my intention for every page of this book. As we get started, be very careful to *not* rush. This isn't a race to the end so you can cross "read *Chasing Cupcakes*" off your to-do list.

While learning can be rushed, changing can't be.

Collecting information is a task. Creating transformation is a *process*. This book isn't here to help you learn about change, it's here to help you **create it.**

I don't know about you, but I've certainly been guilty of flying through a book because the achievement I was after was simply finishing the book. I just wanted to be done so I could move on to the next thing. I gave myself credit for reading books even if I didn't *do* anything with what I learned. I can't help but wonder how many struggles I could have avoided if instead of rushing to learn and move on, I had been patient and committed to the practice of improvement.

I hope you'll learn from my haste. **This is a book about** ***transformation*, not *information*.**

It's not the information you read in these pages that will create change; it's what you choose to *do* with it. I'm not introducing ideas for you to simply read and study; **I'm inviting you to a *practice and process* for *being* the change you want to create.** As you act on what you read, you will step into a future even brighter than the one you imagine.

This is the book I wish existed when I was deep in my own struggle. This offers the support, tactics, and guidance I didn't have.

If you aren't sure how to be stronger than your excuses, this book will provide you with practices to gain strength and certainty.

If you feel overwhelmed by the grip of your old habits and question your ability to break free, this book will give you specific strategies for overcoming the pull of those past patterns.

If you are easily discouraged by what you *can't* do or how far you have to go, this book will help you stay focused on what you *can* do right now.

This book is a tool that will help you win hard moments. It will help you change unconscious patterns and see the truth in the lies (especially the well-intended ones) you tell yourself. It's a companion to help you overcome resistance and create success.

You won't be fighting against yourself but rather working *with* yourself...**creating an operating system of being militantly on your own side.** It will serve as a guide to the joyful pursuit of your best self instead of a battle against your worst self.

There's a big difference between those two approaches.

When you take action on the strategies described in the following pages, you will eliminate the tension between who you are and who you are capable of becoming. You'll shift more easily from fighting those past patterns to living into your potential.

Let me assure you—I won't require or even *recommend* a 180-degree shift in your habits and behaviors. You won't be clearing out your pantry or putting your credit cards in an ice block.

You will create change through *evolution*, not revolution.

I have a feeling you're ready to begin creating change and improving your life. You might be wondering where and how you start.

We'll start by making sure you're doing the right things instead of obsessing over doing all the things right.

MEASURE TWICE, CUT ONCE

"It ain't what you don't know that gets you into trouble. It's what you think you know that just ain't so."

—MARK TWAIN

In any endeavor, while it's important to do your work right, it's *more* important to make sure you're doing the *right work*.

Imagine you're in a boat and suddenly realize there is a hole in the bottom. The boat is taking on water—definitely a problem—what do you do?

Solving the problem is not the same as responding to it.

Responding to the problem might lead you to bail out the water.

Solving the problem requires fixing the hole.

When you bail water, you're dealing with the symptom of the problem, but not the problem itself. When responding to symptoms, your work never ends. **Taking action isn't the same as implementing a solution.**

If you fix the hole in the boat, you've solved the true problem and eliminated the tiring work of bailing.

Lasting results that you achieve *without burnout* require that you identify the problem and solve it. Unfortunately, **most of us exhaust ourselves responding to symptoms of the problem.** This means that we're doing work, and we might even be doing the work right, but we're not doing the right work.

Just the other day, a client reached out to share a struggle. She has a past pattern of wanting to binge eat after work and she wanted help changing that behavior.

She shared with me some of the approaches she'd tried:

meditation, essential oils, hot Epsom salt baths, and exercise. She asked if I had any other suggestions.

Absolutely. **Stop focusing on responding to the problem and start working on solving it.** She doesn't need a *distraction* from thoughts of a binge. That work will be endless! To solve the problem, the right work is **eliminating the appeal of the binge.**

She could do all the things right in creating a distraction, but that's not the right work for her.

As we move forward, the first step we'll take is toward figuring out what the right work is for **you.** To do that, we'll first look at **what's in the way** of the change you're trying to create. In the process, you'll free up all sorts of energy, emotion, and time as you stop doing things that aren't right, aren't necessary, or aren't working.

These next few chapters will lift the veil on your thoughts and choices to expose the root problems behind the symptoms you wrestle with. You'll be amazed at how much more clearly you see your excuses, stories, exceptions, limitations, and struggles as we do that work.

In Part Two, we'll explore strategies for *executing* the work that is right for you. We'll focus on how you can incorporate changes and improvements into your daily life, especially in moments when you're distracted, overwhelmed, stressed, or emotional.

Best-selling author Tim Ferriss says that all that's between you and a better life is a better set of questions. I agree. The magic question is the one that gets great answers from you **and leads you to action, progress, and truth.**

You are likely here because you want some answers. You want to know what to do differently. It's often easier to be told what to do. You might blame your lack of progress on missing information or a need for answers. Though this book won't give you answers, it will help you find them for yourself. It will help you ask better questions and question your current answers—the answers that come up in your life in the form of excuses, doubts, and exceptions.

To help you identify your barriers and make sure you're doing the right work, you'll see there are a number of questions for you to answer in Part One. What you do with these questions will be one of the most transformative steps you take. You have to **ask** the questions. You have to **answer** them and answer them honestly. That might seem obvious, but it's easier said than done. Resist the urge to skim through them. Engage. Participate. See the questions as an opportunity to practice being completely honest with yourself and begin investing your effort in solutions. Finally, you have to **act** on the answer.

Continuing to think the way you've always thought means continuing to act the way you've always acted. These questions are how you'll break through past patterns and create the change you crave.

Don't rush. Don't cut corners.

Once you know the right work for you, we'll move into Part Two and begin focusing on how to execute, overcome excuses, change patterns of behavior, and really make change happen (while continuing to navigate and enjoy your normal, daily life).

Each section within Part Two contains a Creating Change Challenge. Some of these challenges can be completed in a day. Others will suggest a week or more of daily practice.

Take your time and don't lose sight of the fact that learning can be rushed, but changing can't be rushed. Don't forget why you're here and what you're chasing.

We'll wrap up the book with a series of reset reminders. These are a great place to turn when you feel frustrated, defeated, or unmotivated.

I'll summarize how to use this book with something I tell my clients nearly every day:

You will get out of this book what you put into it. The less you put into answering the questions and engaging in the challenges, the less you'll get out of the book. The more you put into it, the more you'll get out of it.

This book is a tool. These tools have the power to change your body, your health, your finances, your relationships, and much more. Like a hammer or a screwdriver, a tool has no value if it sits on a shelf. A tool's value doesn't come from the fact that you know how to use it. The value of a tool comes from what you *do* with it.

While this book contains tools to help you change your life, only you can decide if you'll use them. I hope you won't rob yourself of the opportunity by cutting corners. You deserve more, and more is available to you.

I'm glad you have this book in your hands because it's high time you **end the struggle**, create consistency, build confidence, and live the life you've been longing for. Just picking up this book means change has already started. Things change, right here, right now.

QUESTIONS TO ASK BEFORE WE BEGIN

- What do you want most?
- What do you want to get out of this book?
- What changes do you want to create?

- What is in the way?
- What do you need to let go of?
- What are you afraid to let go of?
- Why are you afraid?
- How will you benefit from letting go of those things?
- What will you do about it today?
- Are you already rushing through these questions?
- Why?
- Do you want to cut corners in the pursuit of creating a life you love?
- What will you do differently while reading this book to ensure that you create changes instead of merely accumulating information?

PART ONE

Breaking Barriers

ONE

The Hard Road

"Why do you always insist on taking the hard road?" one friend asked another. Confused, the friend replied, "Why do you assume I see two roads?"

—UNKNOWN

I was a couple months into writing this book when one of my clients sent me the quote above. Reading it made me realize something important, maybe for the first time.

Often, people who are struggling to change genuinely *don't realize* there is an **easier** way. If they were aware of the easier way, of course they'd choose it!

Typically, when we aren't getting results, we think the only option is to fight harder and for longer.

Fortunately, there *is* a different way.

Here's what I need you to know: the way things have been is not the way they have to continue to be. The road you're on, the road you've traveled up and back and up again for months, years, or maybe even decades...it's *not* the only way.

There is an *easier* way. I know you'll have to see it to believe it, and I'm going to show you. It's not *just* an easier way; it's also more effective and more sustainable. It will end the cycle of doing the work, undoing the work, and doing it over again and again.

One of the primary reasons change feels so hard is that you continue to pour time and energy into strategies that *don't work* for you. They might keep you busy, but they don't solve your underlying problem.

When your path to change is taking you down the hard road, you repeatedly fall short of your expectations. Without a doubt, one of the worst feelings in the world is letting yourself down. It's *hardly* a motivator. It sucks to know you are the primary thing in your own way. Worse yet is not knowing *how* to get out of the way. Very little is more frustrating than waking up *determined* to behave differently, only to find yourself right back in a past pattern you swore you wouldn't choose again.

Those are all hallmarks of the hard road. I recognize it

because I've been there. It's all too familiar to me. I lived on that road for decades and I didn't know any other way. Though I intended for it to be the path to my goals, it brought me to places I really didn't want to be.

Obese. Miserable. Deeply in debt. Depressed. Heading toward divorce.

At my heaviest, if you had asked me what I wanted most in this world, I'd have told you **weight loss**. Hands down. Nothing would have come in a close second. If I could just lose weight, *everything* else would be better. I'd have done *anything* to lose the weight.

Except, it seemed, the work required.

Within hours, sometimes minutes, of thinking about how desperately I wanted to lose weight and planning out all these changes I would make, I'd be eating Hostess cupcakes and Mexican food, followed by a pint of ice cream, all while vowing to do better tomorrow—*and meaning it.* Believing it!

This pattern repeated itself for years. More accurately, I kept *creating* the pattern, day after day, excuse after excuse, wanting a life so different from the one I was choosing.

I used to tell myself that I'd just "get it out of my system."

If I overeat or binge today, I'll get it out of my system for a fresh start tomorrow. I gave in to that lie so quickly that **I didn't allow time for honesty**: it doesn't work. It's not true. It has *never* worked.

I had to stop submitting to the familiar, convenient lies that kept me from creating change. I had to stop shrinking myself into a box of past patterns that I wanted so desperately to step out of. I had to stop living in a cycle of continuous deferment...tomorrow, tomorrow, tomorrow, but never **today.**

I had to stop mortgaging "today" on promises for tomorrow. I was writing checks my future couldn't cash. I was creating habit debt—digging a deeper hole to try to climb out of tomorrow, one destructive, evasive choice at a time.

The price of living that way is high but we aren't stopping to consider what it's costing us.

In order to make the move from the hard path to an easier one, you must first be honest with yourself about what doesn't work or isn't sustainable.

There's a Charlie Munger quote that reminds me of the failing mindset that kept me in a decades-long pattern of choosing an approach that didn't work. He says, "To a man with a hammer, everything looks like a nail."

For me, the solution to every problem was *more willpower!* Willpower was my proverbial hammer—my ineffective approach to solving every problem. Even though it failed me countless times, the approach I kept turning to was the approach that never worked.

I was in an unconscious, unexamined, and unsuccessful habit of valuing intensity over consistency. Working hard instead of working smart.

I was distracted by every new diet and weight loss program. Jumping from one thing to the next was nothing more than a cycle of intensity and inconsistency.

When it came to weight loss, every approach was a variation on the themes of deprivation and restriction.

It never took me where I wanted to go, yet I kept doing it. For years. I was so desperate to change that I didn't stop to reconsider my approach.

Traveling along the easier road requires that you use the power of your brain instead of the intensity of your emotions.

I had to get honest about what didn't work, and you do, too. We'll explore these barriers in more depth in the coming chapters, but for now I want to highlight some of the primary differences between the hard road and the easier one.

As we explore these, look to set aside your ego and resist the urge to defend your patterns and behaviors. The point of these lists isn't to make you feel bad, but to help you identify what doesn't work—without emotion.

Together, through these pages, we are going to lift the veil on the "old way," so we can see through fresh eyes the stories, beliefs, excuses, and patterns that are **slowly eroding the beautiful life that is possible for you.**

We're going to forge a new path that is straighter, simpler, easier, and free from the costly detours of starting, stopping, giving up, giving in, and beginning again.

It will be work, but it won't be as hard as not changing has been. This will be easier than the on-again-off-again, all-or-nothing, I'll-do-better-tomorrow pattern that you've initiated and quit a thousand times before. We'll use our effort to create *lasting* change instead of dancing through the no-change cha-cha. Two steps forward, two steps back, back to the middle, and around again.

No thanks. That pattern is what I not-so-lovingly refer to as "a thousand beginnings and no end in sight."

We're getting off that crazy train. Right now.

Gaining clarity about what *doesn't* work is a prerequisite for creating change and will be a tool you'll use to shift from one approach to the other.

HALLMARKS OF THE HARD ROAD

- Valuing novelty (new approaches) and intensity over consistency.
- Putting off until later what you don't feel like prioritizing today.
- Focusing on your skillset more than your mindset.
- Investing energy in the problem instead of acting on the solution.
- Making yourself a victim of factors outside your control.
- Making decisions based on emotion instead of principle.
- Trying to do everything right instead of focusing on doing the right thing.
- Talking yourself into an excuse instead of talking yourself into progress.
- Focusing more on the journeys and opinions of others than on your own.

No matter how strong some of these habits and patterns

feel, you are free in every moment to choose a different way. Every choice is a chance to make that shift.

HALLMARKS OF THE EASIER ROAD

- Value *consistency* over intensity and novelty.
- Win the moment you're in. Leave yesterday and tomorrow out of it.
- Commit to improving your mindset and perspective every day.
- Invest your energy in creating solutions instead of making a case for the validity of the problem.
- Take advantage of all that is within your control and don't waste energy or place blame on what you can't control.
- Practice principle-based responses instead of emotionally infused reactions.
- Focus on doing the right thing instead of doing all the things right.
- Keep your eyes on your own work. Waste no energy comparing your journey to someone else's.
- Seize every opportunity to break away from past patterns.

You are 100 percent in control of which approach you choose.

No matter how many thousands of times you've made

a choice along the hard road, you're still free to make a decision along the easier road right now. You are free to choose differently in any and every moment. There is absolutely nothing keeping you chained to the hard road.

WHITE KNUCKLES ARE RED FLAGS

Grip something really tight and you'll watch your knuckles turn white as the tension restricts blood flow. As you fight to hold on, your hands give you a visible warning sign: white knuckles.

Do not rely on willpower to create change. White knuckles are red flags.

I was the queen of strict diets. I told myself that more strict meant more effective. I didn't face the full truth that more strict meant less sustainable.

I relied purely on willpower. I remember once doing the infamous HCG diet. For forty days, without exception, I ate just four hundred calories per day and took human chorionic gonadotropin (HCG) drops to stimulate fat-burning during what was essentially a starvation diet. Each day I would eat one grapefruit, one piece of white fish, and half a tomato. Nothing else.

As soon as I deviated from the strict plan, I decided that

my willpower had failed me, and since I was "off," I might as well go *way off*. Sometimes the binge was a day, other times it lasted for weeks. It was a stupid, ineffective approach. It required immeasurable amounts of time, energy, and emotion. Most importantly, *it did not work.*

I felt like I was constantly fighting against myself, and when you're fighting against yourself, you always lose.

This fight, this desperate grip, the tension you generate to avoid losing control—I see it all the time when people are trying to create change.

It's resistance, resentment, discipline, and willpower.

I call it white-knuckle willpower. It is a hallmark of the hard road.

It's you against yourself.

You against your habits.

You against what you want.

You against temptation and past patterns.

Yes, restriction and white-knuckle willpower are *one* option for change, but not the only one. They're not the easiest option, not the most sustainable option, and certainly not the most pleasant option.

I get it. Willpower is very "in" right now. Everyone wants to be tough and hardcore. We beat ourselves up when we drop the ball and wake up intending to be more strict in the days ahead.

There is no badge of honor for misery. There is no award granted for toughness.

Seeing this journey as your mind against your body or your past against your future overlooks a critical truth: there's only one team. **You are doing this work for yourself.**

If you're fighting against yourself and you convince yourself that there are two sides, you can't ever win.

Don't choose that perspective.

Forget the intense, all-in, white-knuckle willpower lifestyle overhaul you've been considering or wrestling with. Let go of the worry about how you'll stay on track next weekend. **Instead, choose to be intentional about the progress you're committing to each day.**

You are not stuck. Your temptations, impulses, and past

patterns do not have more control than you do. In fact, those temptations, impulses, and past patterns have absolutely no control. *Only* you do.

When you feel unfocused or overwhelmed, take a look at the mental models characteristic of the hard road and the easy road and **challenge yourself to just make one choice from the perspective of the easier road.**

That's all it ever takes! You are always just a few great choices away from feeling better, building momentum, and creating the change you crave.

QUESTIONS TO ASK

- What are some of the ways you're operating along the hard road?
- What would it look like to make change easier today?
- What is life on the hard road costing you?
- In what ways are you willing and able to practice making things easier?
- Until you create change, what will you continue to miss out on?
- What is the difference between working with yourself and working against yourself?
- How can you be militantly on your own side today?

TWO

Spinning Your Wheels

"Sometimes we fail so slowly we think we are succeeding."

—GARY KELLER

Often, we judge ourselves based on our intentions instead of holding ourselves accountable to our results. Because we're *thinking* about what we want, because we have the *desire* to change and we *plan* to do so, we give ourselves credit for trying even when our efforts aren't producing results.

You can see this unproductive pattern all around you.

Frustrated with how his tax dollars were being spent, a California man went to his town meeting to get some answers. He took the floor to ask why the city seemed more invested in regulations related to motorized scooter use than in the growing problems of homelessness and drug abuse. The town representative explained that this wasn't the case at all. In fact, the representative informed the man, the town actually spends ten times more on homelessness than on scooter covenant enforcement.

To that, the concerned taxpayer replied, "Sir, I'm from the business world. We judge progress based on outputs, not inputs. Don't tell me how much money you're spending. I want you to tell me how the money you're spending is making a difference."

This town representative was giving credit for effort without addressing what matters most: What results does the effort produce?

When you're trying to create change, it's *not* time to argue for how hard you're trying, how far you've come, how much better you are than you used to be, how healthy you eat, or how much less you spend. Those factors simply aren't relevant.

Don't let the investment cloud your awareness of its impact.

Don't allow yourself to overvalue your investment of time, money, desire, effort, or thought. Don't overlook the lack of impact that investment is having on your end goal.

I am all for appreciating the progress you've made in the past, but it doesn't have a place in *justifying* the lack of progress you're presently making.

Don't let past success become a barrier to present and future progress.

Don't focus so much on your effort and intent that you lose sight of whether or not it's producing results.

Stay closely connected to what matters most: *Is it working?* Are you where you want to be? Are you moving in the right direction? Is your pace acceptable to you?

When the answer is no, it's time to change. In fact, when the answer is anything other than an immediate and emphatic "yes!" it's time to change. Don't continue to waste time and energy justifying or validating your lack of progress. Simply change something.

How much easier would the pursuit of your goals be if you stopped putting so much effort into strategies that aren't working?

ARE YOU GETTING SOMEWHERE?

A couple years ago, I was moving from my loft in New Hampshire to a new apartment in Massachusetts. It was an unseasonably warm day in February and the massive snowbanks were softening.

My mom's boyfriend came by in his pickup truck to help with the move. He backed his truck as close to my porch as it would go, right into the melting snow.

Channeling a more patient, less bossy version of myself, I bit my tongue and didn't verbalize my nervousness about parking his truck in the snow. We didn't have a lot of time and I certainly didn't feel like digging him out if the truck got stuck.

We loaded up the cars and got ready to leave. As I pulled out in my Jeep, I heard the unmistakable sound of tires spinning. No, they weren't mine. Yup, Bob's truck was stuck in the snow.

The engine was revving, his tires were spinning, and with every passing second, he was digging a deeper hole in the snow.

The harder he pressed the accelerator, the worse it got. Dirt and snow spit out from under the furious tires, painting the bright-white house a soft mud color.

Awesome.

He'd pull forward an inch and throttle the gas again. Nothing.

Back up an inch and repeat. Nothing.

Same approach, same results.

If points were awarded for effort, he might get some. But points for progress? None.

You can keep up the effort, but if you aren't going anywhere, you won't get anywhere.

You have to try something different—something that *works*.

Effort and progress are two very different things. They're absolutely not interchangeable.

Too many of us stay in those proverbial "tire tracks" for decades. We throttle our effort and do the most obvious thing, even if it isn't getting us anywhere. We back up an inch or two, scoot forward an inch or two, give it all we've got, but don't get where we're trying to go. Then we tell ourselves a story about how hard we're trying.

We're in such a rush to "try" that we don't slow down to

evaluate if what we're trying is actually moving us in the right direction.

Be careful of giving yourself points for effort when the effort isn't creating the change you crave.

INFORMATION ISN'T TRANSFORMATION

One of the most common ways we spin our wheels and make change harder than it needs to be is by valuing learning over doing—giving ourselves credit for gathering information.

You'd better believe I considered writing my first book about hormones or fat loss—people flock to those kinds of books—but I don't believe we need more information.

At 350 pounds, I already knew about (and had tried) every diet under the sun. I wasn't in need of more information on what to eat or not eat. I knew I wasn't making great choices consistently. All the options were just one of many ways I talked myself out of consistency. Learning felt productive and it was infinitely easier than *doing*.

The majority of the time, we know more than enough to create change. **Piling on more information is not the path to creating transformation.** In fact, accumulating more information can be a barrier to change! We can know *so* much that we actually feel overwhelmed by all the options. I see a lot of people who are addicted to learning. What they need is a healthy dose of *doing!*

Recently, I had a client ask if I would provide transcripts of our coaching webinars. She explained that she's a visual learner. She likes to underline and rewrite important ideas and phrases.

Makes sense. That's how we're taught to learn in school. Accumulate information. Memorize.

But, I'll tell you the same thing I told her.

You aren't here to learn. You're here to *change.*

You don't need to take notes; you need to take action.

Learning things you could change and why you should change them is entirely different from *actively participating in creating change.*

Think about it—you don't become a great basketball player by studying the sport, memorizing statistics, and drawing plays. Knowing a lot about basketball is not the same thing as being a great basketball player. You cannot become a great player on the sidelines, learning about the sport.

You become a great player by playing—by getting off the sidelines and making plays, over and over, learning from *your* experience, not from someone else's theory. You need to spend time taking the shots and learning from each attempt.

For all of us, creating change demands that we get off the sidelines and into the game.

Tim Elmore refers to this learning trap as "artificial maturity" and explains that artificial maturity is the byproduct of two colliding realities:

1. Overexposure to information
2. Underexposure to experience

That right there basically sums up one of the massive barriers to creating change. Too much information, not enough consistent practice.

Fortunately, this is something over which you have total control! **You can choose, today and every day, in your next moment and any moment, to practice** *living* **what you know and** *learning from doing* **instead of accumulating more information.**

It's not a mystery, this process of creating change. We act like we're confused and overwhelmed, when in reality,

we're just not taking action. That's where most of our best answers will come from anyway: our own action.

It's time to prioritize action over information.

I made this information-over-implementation mistake in the grandest fashion.

I got a bachelor's degree in nutrition! At my heaviest, I was also pursuing a master's degree in nutrition! I was working for a major hospital system as an obesity-prevention specialist while I was tipping the scales over 350 pounds.

I was desperate for solutions and I thought I'd find them accumulating more information. I didn't.

Knowing what to do doesn't help at all when you have a habit of justifying why today isn't the day to do the work— convincing yourself that tomorrow holds some promise today doesn't.

Knowing what to do doesn't help at all when you convince yourself that this one thing won't make a difference anyway.

It's not about how much you know. It's about what you consistently do. It's not about taking notes; it's about taking action.

While I love the fact that we live in this age of easy information, I also think it's a big part of why we're on the hard road. We want to know more—as much as we can—and we mistakenly believe that if we just keep listening to the information, to the motivation, to the encouragement, one day it will click.

That's not how it works.

All this information consumption can backfire. **Learning feels productive.** Psychologically, it can feel as satisfying, in the short term, as *actually* taking action.

Let's say your goal is weight loss. When you listen to a podcast on weight loss, you feel like you've done something good for your health. You feel motivated! Informed! You prioritized learning. Check! Pat on head.

But, if you haven't *done* anything with what you learned, if you haven't taken *action* that moves you toward the change you want, what you're feeling is a false sense of accomplishment that will hold you back from true progress.

You check the box of understanding and move right along without ever implementing, without ever practicing and making what you learned your own.

Even if *you* don't experience that false sense of accomplishment or productivity, you might feel something worse: **the crushing disappointment of the widening gap between what you know and what you're actually doing.** You'll bounce from approach to approach, plan to plan—the journey with a thousand beginnings and not an end in sight.

It's time to stop spinning your wheels. Set your ego aside and refuse to argue for your time, effort, and intention. Keep it simple: Is it working?

QUESTIONS TO ASK

- Is your approach working?
- What results are your efforts producing?
- Where are there gaps between what you know and what you do?
- What will you do to close those gaps this week?
- Where are you attracted to accumulating knowledge?
- How can you use some of that time and energy on action?

THREE

Check Your Ego

"You are the teacher you have been waiting for.

You can end your own suffering."

—BYRON KATIE

You are the problem.

You are the reason you haven't yet created the change you crave.

Before you get defensive and begin making a case for why I'm wrong and it's not your fault (it's work stress, your menopausal metabolism, family dynamics, or absolutely anything else), take a breath. This is one of the most important starting points for creating change and getting out of your own way.

When you realize you've been one of the biggest barriers to your own change and you take full responsibility, you put yourself in a place of power.

When you don't take responsibility and instead place blame on other people and things, you strip yourself of your power.

This is *good* news because you are also the solution.

You are powerful beyond measure. You already have what it takes to create change. I refuse to endorse any other perspective and I hope you choose to agree.

You must stop convincing yourself that you're smaller than your circumstances, because you're not. Your circumstances do not have more power than you do.

Your past patterns are simply more practiced, more familiar, and maybe more comfortable, but they have no power, except that which you give them through your perspective. *You* have the power. You *are* the power.

There is no circumstance or habit that removes your power to choose a different way of being.

Your circumstances don't make you less able to choose change or be changed. There is no circumstance or habit that removes your *ability* to take impeccable care of yourself.

We are going to start *living into that truth* and becoming **vibrant change agents**, one moment at a time.

It's going to require some serious ego checking, but don't worry, I'll help with that.

To step into this new truth about your ever-present ability to create change in any moment, **you'll need to set aside all your frustration and disappointment about past attempts and patterns.** No, seriously, that's a requirement. When your past takes up too much space in your perspective, it crowds out all your present potential.

Don't argue for why you can't or how hard it is. As I'll continue to remind you in the coming chapters, you must give your energy to what you *can* do, not to what you can't. You must stop participating in the problem so you can bring about the solution.

There's no growth or change available to you when you are committed to the problem or convinced of the impossibility.

It's time to go exclusively *forward*...powerfully, intelligently, and enthusiastically **forward**.

As Chicken Soup creator Jack Canfield reminds us, "Work is required. Suffering is optional."

Self-improvement is a gift, not a curse. It's a blessing, not a burden. It represents giving yourself something, not taking something away.

Let's not deny or overlook the fact that there is a gap between your *understanding* that you *can* create change and the *work* it's going to take to create it. In the gap lives the big, overwhelming question of "How?" In the gap lies doubt, rising from those past patterns we're not giving our emotion to any longer.

It's natural to feel overwhelmed or skeptical. It's true that there are hundreds of options and unlimited approaches. You're also probably thinking through everything you've tried before, every time you've dropped the ball, everything you've read and heard, what your friends have done, what you saw on Facebook, the goals you want to accomplish, your fear of failure, what is going on in your life, and your social obligations, preferences, and lifestyle. Whoa. It's a lot. **When you put all that together, it's a recipe for doing *nothing at all* because the "*something*" isn't clear.** See that trap. Refuse to step in it again.

Since complexity is the enemy of execution, we're going to keep it really simple. You might think you need more time, more information, more support, or more willpower to create these changes, but you don't.

You have everything you need.

Every day, I get emails from people who declare, "My problem is cravings. My problem is alcohol. My problem is snacking. My problem is inconsistency."

I see it differently. **It's not your problem; it's your practice.**

I respond to those emails by asking, "What does your practice look like?" If you've told me that your problem is snacking, I ask, "What does your snacking practice look like?"

It looks a lot like the problem, doesn't it?

Precisely.

Your practice is what creates the problem.

Your practice is what will create the solution.

Are you practicing the problem?

Are you practicing solutions?

Which do you practice more?

Don't stray too far from these simple questions.

If you feel like your problem is snacking after dinner, and you eat every night after dinner, your practice is reinforcing the problem.

You don't have a snacking problem; you have a *snacking practice*.

Similarly, whatever your problem is, that is also your *opportunity* to practice the solution.

YOU (ALREADY) HAVE WHAT YOU NEED

Just the other day, I had a phone call with a client. I asked her **what she wants more of that she doesn't have right now.** She explained that she's disappointing herself with her food choices. She starts the day strong but always ends the day overeating and overindulging.

I repeated the question. "What do you want more of in your life?"

Don't tell me about the problem. Let's talk about the solution.

"Control," she said. "I need more control."

"Jane," I replied, "you already have all the control you'll ever have and you have all the control you'll ever need."

There is a difference between not *having* control and not *taking* control. There is a difference between not having control and not *being* controlled in your thoughts and choices.

You don't need more control, which is great news because you can't *get* more. You *can* leverage it better. You can use it differently. Let's be clear: you have the same amount of control over your food choices or your financial choices as everyone else has, and you have all the control you could ever need.

You can probably relate to this on many levels—not taking control of spending choices, not taking control of projects at home, or not taking control of your food choices.

This came up recently with a group of my clients. Every week I do live Q and A webinars, and on one of the last webinars, someone asked, "Elizabeth, how do you respond when you have sugar cravings? What are your go-tos when your cravings are out of control?"

My cravings aren't ever out of control, and neither are yours.

They are within my control because I hold the power to choose. The cravings do not. I am in control of my choices in each moment, whether cravings are a factor or not. So what do I choose? Nothing. I choose nothing. Every moment I have a craving, I have a chance to rewire my past pattern of responding to them and letting them influence my decisions. The feeling of desire doesn't win. I choose control. I take control. I am controlled.

It's both a perspective and a practice.

Can I convince myself that my cravings are in control? Of course. Does that make it true? No.

That's the huge paradigm shift. My cravings don't control my food choices. I do. It doesn't mean I don't ever indulge—I do. But my cravings don't make those decisions. I do. I am in control and so are you.

My past doesn't define me and neither do my patterns; **my present practice does.**

I'm free to create a new practice, one that serves me, in any and every moment. So are you.

When you feel like you're lacking control, recognize that in that moment, you are letting a familiar and favored reality dominate your thoughts. It's a choice you are making, subconsciously or consciously.

There's a different way you can choose. You are free to practice a different response. You are free to be *changed* in that moment. You are free to *be* change in that moment.

There is a dramatic difference between hoping for change and choosing change in the moment you're in.

Every choice is a chance to be a better version of yourself. A more disciplined version. A more thoughtful version. A bolder version. A more focused version.

You have everything it takes to make that choice. Stop telling yourself that you aren't there yet. **Don't submit to the lie of tomorrow.** Instead, choose to be the change now.

Change never needs to wait until tomorrow. You don't need a plan. You don't need a program. You don't need to get anything out of your system. **You simply need to win this moment.**

This, right here, this next moment, is your next chance to change.

You already have everything you need.

QUESTIONS TO ASK

- What do you want more of in your life?
- What past problems do you focus on?
- In what ways are you practicing the problem?
- How will you practice the solution?
- What will you do today to practice the change you desire?
- In your life and circumstances, what does it look like to take control?
- How will you practice this in the next forty-eight hours?

FOUR

Transformation Is Now

"Presence is where the payoff is. Just be with what is going on in front of you. The next right step comes from that place."

—DANIELLE LAPORTE

Change can be overwhelming. It can feel like there is *endless* work between where you are now and where you want to be. On top of that, when you're looking at the changes you want to make through a filter of fear, doubt, and past experiences, it can seem like an impossible journey—one you're not yet equipped to make. Maybe it feels like you've already failed or that your destination is a far-off place you might never see.

Most people think that change is something you pursue.

That perspective convinces us that change is in the future—that it's not *here* yet. That's simply not true.

Transformation is *not* a journey you pursue. Transformation is **now**. Change happens in any moment you choose it.

Transformation is a decision, not a destination. It is an opportunity summoned by your ever-present ability to choose. It's here in *every* moment.

Tom Peters explains this brilliantly when he says that excellence is not an aspiration; **excellence is the next five minutes.**

Excellence is your next conversation. It's your next email. It's your next procedure. It's your next meal. It's your next workout. Excellence, like transformation, is an opportunity that exists, no matter what your next five minutes entails.

Transformation is a present choice, not a future outcome. You don't have to earn it, you have to choose it, and every choice is a chance.

You're not alone if you've been quick to let yourself off the hook because, quite frankly, there's always tomorrow. You're not alone if you've justified a choice with the reassuring thought that you can always start later. You're not alone if you can't identify with the change you want to create because it's not *here* yet. It hasn't happened. You're not *there* yet. You haven't earned it.

When you plan to do better tomorrow, you miss the chances (choices) in front of you today.

When you see change as something that exists in the future, what you don't see clearly is the opportunity to choose change *now*. You don't take responsibility for the work that presents itself today because who and how you want to be is out on the horizon of your life.

"Transformation is now" means you can *be* different right now. You *need* to be. This is when change happens. This next moment is your chance. This next choice is your opportunity.

No moment can be dismissed. No choice is too small to make a difference.

NOW VERSUS TODAY

I recently worked with a professional copywriter to help me create a new tagline for the *Primal Potential* podcast. I explained that it's not really a show about hormones or nutrition—it's about living into and up to your highest potential—and I wanted the tagline of the show to reflect that.

As I threw out ideas, he'd repeat them back so I could hear what they sounded like. Sometimes he'd adjust them a little, suggesting a different word or phrase.

I enthusiastically proclaimed, "Transformation is now!"

Sounding unconvinced and a little confused, he replied, "Transformation is today."

I cringed. "No. Nope. That's totally different. Now and today don't send the same message."

He didn't get it.

I explained, "If you tell me that transformation is today, the best response you'll get from me is an eye roll. I don't have time for this huge idea today. I have to work, I have to squeeze in a workout, my inbox is out of control and I have no idea what I'm doing for dinner tonight. Transformation is definitely not today." It's asking too much of me. It's asking for more than I feel I can give.

At *best*, I'd be skeptical and dismissive. At worst, I'd be annoyed and shut down.

However, "transformation is now" reminds me that I can *be* different in **every** moment. **It's not something I have to make time for.** The time already exists. It's something I can choose as I go through *any* day. The opportunities for transformation exist in the choices I'm already making. I either choose change or I choose more of the same. "Transformation is now" means that as I go about my normal day, transformation is simply acting like the best version of myself, or even a *better* version of myself in one, two, or all of my mundane moments. Change is available to me in *every* choice.

"Transformation is now" reminds me that I can choose change right now by drinking water instead of more coffee. It reminds me that I can choose change right now by resisting distractions instead of submitting to them. "Transformation is now" reminds me that the next time I open the refrigerator is a chance to be changed.

You, too, can choose to **be** change in this moment. And the next moment. In every moment. Excellence is the next five minutes.

YOU HAVE TO BE HERE, NOW

To embrace the opportunity of change that exists in all your moments, you have to actually be *in* the moments as they happen. I don't know about you, but quite frequently,

I catch myself somewhere else. Maybe I'm thinking about something that happened earlier that day or something going on later.

A boyfriend of mine helped me see this play out in real time. We were at the driving range, hitting golf balls. I am not a golfer; it was probably my fifth trip to a driving range in as many years. As he made solid contact, swing after swing, driving the ball straight down the fairway, I struggled. Often, I'd miss the ball altogether. After hearing me mutter "Damnit!" a few dozen times, he stepped back to watch me. Walking back to his clubs, he said, "Keep your head down. Don't look down range before you've even hit the ball. You're missing what's right at your feet because you're not looking. Head down."

I took his advice and, sure enough, it worked. I started making contact with the ball. That one simple adjustment not only produced immediate results, it also felt easier!

As we drove home, I thought about the broader application of my free golf lesson.

When you're looking ahead (or behind), you can't see the opportunity at your feet. If you want to go somewhere, you can't overlook the chance for progress that's right in front of you.

Tim Ferriss shares a similar lesson in his book *Tribe of Mentors*. While training with a famous tennis pro and struggling to make consistent contact with the ball, the pro instructed Ferriss to focus exclusively on **the point of impact**. Instead of looking at where he wanted the ball to go, he was only to focus on the moment the ball hit his racket.

Like my experience at the driving range, focusing on the point of impact immediately improved his game and it felt easier!

"Transformation is now" is another way to remind yourself to focus on the point of impact: the moment you're in right now and what you can do in it to create progress.

There's a great quote from author Danielle Laporte: "**Presence is where the payoff is.** Just be with what's going on in front of you. The next right step comes from that place."

Deciding that **transformation is now** is where the payoff is. It's the *only* place the payoff is. Be with the opportunity for change and growth that is right in front of you right now. Every choice is a chance.

What is the best next choice you can make?

Don't keep rehashing the last five years. Let it go. It's gone. You don't need to stress about how far you have to go. That won't help. In fact, it will probably hurt you and obscure your ability to make progress as it takes your attention away from your opportunity to choose change right now.

Do the work that exists for you in *this* moment. That's all you have to do. That's all there *is* to do. Be with what's going on in front of you. Don't justify this moment based on the past and don't disregard it on future promises. Just be here now.

Remember how we said we'd keep it simple? There's nothing simpler than **winning the moment you're in**.

Release the past and stay out of the future. Be here, now.

As powerfully simply as this idea is, I need to caution you about a gross misuse of the notion that every choice is a chance.

It's **not** permission to blow off every immediate opportunity for progress because, hey, *there's always next time*. It is not meant to give you an unending pass on the choice in front of you right now.

Quite the opposite, actually. "Every choice is a chance"

instructs you to capitalize on each moment, *not* defer to the next.

The only moment that matters, the only moment that can change your life, is the one you're currently in.

If "every choice is a chance" feels like a cop-out, you're doing it wrong. Check yourself. Win the moment you're in.

To embrace the opportunity presented by the idea that transformation is now, you'll have to stop focusing on what you can't do, what you don't want to do, or what you've already tried. All of those thoughts will distract you from what you can do now—from how you can choose change in this moment.

The only place you have *any* power or impact is now. It's the only moment that is real. The past can't be changed and the future isn't an option until it is the present.

Stop putting off until tomorrow what you are able to do today.

The pattern of delay offers zero opportunity for progress. Pushing off your goals or the work required to achieve them until tomorrow, next week, when work slows down, the kids go back to school, the first of the year, or any other time is to dismiss the fact that you can create change right now. Excellence is your next five minutes.

There is something you can do today. Do it.

Of course, it's easy to justify submitting to temptation, especially when you tell yourself that you'll make a different choice tomorrow.

I have no doubt that your intentions are good. I'm quite certain you believe that pledge when you make it.

But every choice is a chance to break that failing pattern.

This habit of tomorrow ensures that you won't make progress. It ensures that you'll continue to struggle. It guarantees that you won't create the consistency needed to create and maintain lasting change.

That operating system of "later" teaches you to ignore the only opportunity that exists in reality to change: now.

If you quit today, it's going to be that much easier for you to quit tomorrow. If you talk yourself out of action today, it's going to be that much easier to talk yourself out of action tomorrow. If you persist today, it will be that much easier to persist tomorrow!

Do you ever hit the snooze button on your alarm clock?

Most people do. They set their alarm for a specific time and then choose the comfort of the moment over their previous night's intentions. Snooze. They kick off their day by breaking a promise they've made to themselves and choosing comfort over integrity. They've rehearsed, countless times, the belief that what they want *now* matters more than what they want *most*.

They value staying in bed (temptation of the moment) over keeping their word (getting up when the alarm goes off).

Sure, it's innocent enough when you still make it to work on time, but I want you to see that it's the operating system of "later" that is the problem. It's also the opportunity to create change.

Hitting snooze is practicing the same pattern you choose when you tell yourself you'll work out, eat cleaner, or update your budget *tomorrow*.

If we had to give that behavior a voice, it would say, "Why do it now if I can do it later? I'm not in the mood to change now. My comfort matters more than my growth."

Why go to the gym today when I can make a case to go tomorrow?

Why skip dessert today if I promise to eat cleaner tomorrow?

Why make that phone call I planned to make today if I can do it later?

It's insidious and impairs every area of life it touches.

I realize that it's cliché to say that today is a gift, but it is. It's an opportunity. Discipline isn't going to be easier tomorrow. Change won't be easier tomorrow.

It will never be easier than it is now. Now is your chance.

I read once that the cost of change today is a bargain compared to what it will cost you tomorrow. The more time you let go by without creating that change, the harder it will be when you finally get around to it.

Change will never be easier than it is today. Any voice in your head that tells you otherwise exists only to keep you in your comfort zone. Break out.

Have you ever seen those signs on the highway that advertise apartment complexes? They say something like, "*If you lived here, you'd be home by now!*"

My friend, if you hadn't passed up so many thousands

of opportunities to change, your struggle would be over now.

Don't let that discourage you. Let it remind you of the power in each moment so you reconsider passing them off and opting for later. Every choice is a chance. Every moment is a step on your journey to your goal.

You are capable of seizing the opportunities that exist today to create change. You can make every choice you make bring you closer to the life you want. Or you can add stress and prolong the struggle by continuing to delay.

What if, just for one day, you seized every single moment and every single choice as a chance to move in the direction of your goals?

Are you willing to try that?

Did you just consider having that day be tomorrow instead of today?

No! TODAY!

Be on the lookout for moments when you put off change. Now is always the most important moment. Now is always *your* moment.

What if, for the rest of *this* day, you seized every single moment and every single choice as a chance to move in the direction of your goals?

When you're ordering at a restaurant, use it as an opportunity to move toward your goal.

When you're cleaning your kitchen or grocery shopping, seize that very moment as a chance to act or think in a way that moves you toward your goals.

Every single choice is a chance and every day is full of chances that are disguised as choices.

How will you seize them?

What can you do today to practice becoming a **now** person?

Wash your dish as soon as you finish it.

Fold the laundry as soon as you take it out of the dryer.

Make that phone call you've been putting off.

Make the best choice at dinner instead of pledging to do better tomorrow.

Pay the bill that's been sitting on the counter for a week.

Train yourself to be on the lookout for these opportunities to avoid delay.

Change is a result of what you do now, not what you intend to do tomorrow.

When you think of your goal as someplace you're going to later, you can always delay the trip by an hour or day. But change isn't someplace you travel to. It's a place you create and your best chance is now.

Stop convincing yourself that there's no harm in later. It's just not true. It's terribly harmful. It's about more than procrastination. The delay you give in to is actually creating an outcome you don't want.

Hesitation is the cornerstone of mediocrity.

Delay isn't a victimless crime. **You are the victim.** Your health, happiness, confidence, and peace of mind are all on the line.

Go through each day with your eyes wide open, seeing every choice you make as an opportunity to create change in the moment you're in. It's the most important time.

QUESTIONS TO ASK

- What are three opportunities you can seize today to create transformation?
- How will you remind yourself to choose transformation every day this week?
- What change have you been putting off that you can take action on today?
- Where do you have opportunities for improvement in your actions, thoughts, or reactions today?
- How will you practice intentionally redirecting your thoughts and attention to the present moment?
- Are you practicing being the best version of yourself?
- What are you putting off?
- What can you do today that will make tomorrow easier?

FIVE

Barriers to Change

"Writing is easy. All you have to do is cross out the wrong words."

—MARK TWAIN

The most effective approach to removing the barriers between yourself and the change you crave can be found in these words from Mark Twain. The barrier to great writing is very much like the barriers to progress in our lives. We don't need to add more to the story. We need to remove what's in the way of it flowing freely.

Best-selling author Tim Ferriss does a great job describing how he uses this idea in his own writing. As he edits his books, he's looking to identify and remove anything that causes the story to drag. Extra words, redundant stories, and unnecessary phrases can slow it down. They get in the way and take away from flow and momentum. A great book eliminates all the parts of the story that aren't strong.

The same is true in your life. To make progress and create a life you love living, you have to identify and remove what slows you down, adds to drag, and gets in the way of your goals. You have to find "the wrong words" and cross them out.

Our progress is thwarted more by what *shouldn't be* in our thoughts or actions but *is* than by what *isn't* there but should be.

Though a common approach to creating change is to add more (do more), the easier, more *effective* approach to creating change is to eliminate the thoughts and behaviors that aren't working.

The famous artist Michelangelo captured this idea in the most beautiful word picture. When asked about his work carving the massive statue of David from a single block of marble, he said, "I saw the angel in the marble and carved until I set him free."

He removed everything that *wasn't* part of the magnificent form of David.

You can relax the perspective that you need to add something new that will work. Instead, remove all that *doesn't*.

In most cases, it's *your thoughts and your stories about the past and the problem* that create the most drag in your life. They consume so much of your attention that you don't have much time or energy left to engage with the solution.

As we do this work, you won't be complicating your life; you'll be simplifying it.

While a lot of people approach change by pledging to eat less or move more, what's preventing progress is the "I'll start tomorrow" story and the endless excuses. It doesn't matter *what* you plan to add when you repeatedly dismiss opportunities to do the work by telling yourself, "Just this once...it won't hurt." It doesn't matter how badly you want to achieve your goal when, in frustration or fatigue, you manufacture a story about how you don't even care.

These are the words you'll begin crossing out. These are the barriers to change that drag you down and hold you back.

I try to identify and remove these barriers daily by asking and answering one simple question: *What can I release that is no longer serving me?*

Some days my answer is "Stressing out about other people's opinions!" Other days, it's as simple as "Sugar."

If you already doubt your ability to remove these barriers because your behavior patterns feel so deeply engrained that they're practically automatic, I have a request to make: **stop fueling your doubt with your attention and emotion.**

Stop talking yourself into the problem. **These barriers have no power of their own.** They only have the power and influence you *give* them. You give them power and influence when you *choose* them. You give them power and influence when you argue for them.

When you argue for your limitations, you remain restricted by them. When you argue for your limitations, you get to keep them.

Until you identify and remove your barriers, you are essentially trying to drive down the highway of change with your parking brake on. No matter how hard you try, you'll be fighting against a strong current.

Let's explore this parking brake analogy for a minute.

Imagine we're in the car together. You're in the driver's seat and I'm sitting beside you. We're merging onto the highway and the engine is revving hard. You are grimacing. You've got the pedal to the metal but we're *barely* moving. Something is definitely wrong. It's clear that both you and the car are struggling. It's harder than it should be.

You press the gas pedal harder, but the car only resists you more.

Other cars are flying by; they don't appear to be struggling. You're the slowest one on the road.

You're frustrated. Your leg is tense. You're pressing the gas with all your strength, to no avail.

I put my hand on your arm and gently say, "Hey, ease up. Your parking brake is on. Take a second to pull over and release it."

Irritated, you reply, "I don't have time to stop!"

You press the gas harder. More effort but still no results.

I'm just curious. What would happen if you *did* make that time for the short pause to pull to the side and release the brake?

Everything would *immediately* get easier. Though you

might lose a few seconds in the short term, you'd quickly make it up with the newfound ease and efficiency. You wouldn't have to work as hard. The car wouldn't have to work as hard. It wouldn't resist you. You wouldn't be frustrated anymore.

No matter how much willpower you have, it won't overcome the drag of the parking brake. And while you can come up with a million strategies to make the car go faster, the only *effective* one is to release the brake to remove the source of the drag.

Imagine I'm still sitting beside you in the car, my hand gently on your arm. "Hey, you're working so hard. You want this badly, but I see the problem. Your parking brake is engaged."

You might feel like you can't stop pushing, even if it's not working. You might even feel a bit afraid of what might happen if you take your foot off the gas.

But, my friend, you don't have time *not* to. You're making this harder than it needs to be. Until you release it, until you remove the resistance, you'll grow increasingly frustrated and you'll exhaust yourself with futile effort. Right now, you're wasting a lot of energy and time. There's a much better way.

Author Seth Godin reinforces this simply. "Staying on the wrong bus won't make it the right bus." Sure wish he had told me that twenty years ago!

Sticking with an ineffective approach won't make it an effective one. Don't fear changing your approach; the only thing to fear is continuing to do something that doesn't work.

The most important thing you're going to have to change is your mind.

Of course, we all have external barriers, including time limitations, financial limitations, and physical limitations, but *our biggest barriers are the ones we have constructed in our own minds*.

You are confined primarily by the walls *you* have built.

It's time to take them down.

As I remind my clients when they're struggling to create change: **white knuckles are red flags**. If you feel like you're fighting against yourself, don't resist the problem; **move toward it with curiosity**. You have a choice. You can work with yourself or you can work against yourself. Instead of grimacing and fighting against yourself the way you'd be fighting against a car with the parking brake on, work with your mind and your body. Don't just slap on layer after layer of behavior change. Ask yourself some questions so you can identify the real problem and begin to untangle it.

What's in the way?

What's making this hard?

What's the resistance to this change?

What can I do about it?

Slow down and evaluate what's causing the drag.

You won't reach your potential, create the change you crave, or live the life you're capable of until you remove your barriers.

As we hone in on your personal barriers to change, you will see, as I did, as so many of my clients have, that you won't just make faster, easier progress toward your goal, but that *every* aspect of your life will improve.

When "delay" is no longer your operating system, you'll find that you are more productive at home and at work—

allowing yourself to achieve more across every area of your life—and more quickly!

I've seen clients lose massive amounts of weight, launch businesses, get promotions, become more attentive parents, save their marriage, find the love of their life, pay down mountains of debt, and much more.

Identifying how these barriers impede progress in your life and working to remove them will transform your mindset, attitude, energy, body, relationships, finances, career, and health.

With these barriers removed, the positive changes you make will no longer meet concrete resistance.

When you finally focus on the real barriers to success instead of jumping from new habit to new habit, it will be like seeing with clear eyes for the very first time—the mental pollution of doubt and excuses will lift.

"It's very hard to grow because it's difficult to let go of the models of ourselves in which we've invested so heavily."

—RAM DASS

Pause for a second and think about ideas and limitations that hold you back. Consider all aspects of your life.

Do you define yourself as an all-or-nothing person?

Do you believe you're overemotional?

Do you describe yourself as someone who starts strong but never finishes?

As you begin to consider your limitations and the barriers you've built in your mind, I have some very important words of caution: **don't believe everything you think.**

A major barrier to behavior change is **clinging to beliefs that are familiar but not true.** Though perhaps they were true in the *past*, the only reason they feel true now is because you still subscribe to them. You believe them. You endorse them with your thoughts and fuel them with your attention. You reinforce and empower them with your choices.

Some of the hardest work you'll do in the process of creating change is **letting go of these beliefs that reflect where you've been, but not where you're going.** They aren't relevant anymore. If you choose to live in the past, your future will look just like it. You have to let those beliefs go.

You must refuse to fuel those thoughts and ideas with your intentions and actions. Who you have been doesn't limit who you can choose to *be* today. What you have done in the past doesn't limit what you're free to do today.

Last spring, I had the amazing privilege of spending the weekend with a handful of people from the Primal Potential Masters Club. One afternoon, I was listening to one of my friends share that she wants to be strong—both mentally and physically stronger than she is now. At the same time, she was expressing a lot of doubt and uncertainty. For at least ten minutes, she spoke about the past, how she had drifted, given up, and let herself down, repeatedly. She talked in great detail about the excuses she has given in to, the ways she talked herself out of her best effort, and her ongoing disappointment that she hasn't made more progress.

Though she had this desire to become a strong woman, she was very much attached to the story of how things had been in the past. She was arguing for a past pattern of weakness and pulling those patterns forward into the present, placing a negative filter over an otherwise blank slate of a day. She was more emotionally invested in the problem than the solution. She was more connected to her past pattern of weakness than her present ability to be strong.

There was total incongruence between her **intention** (to be strong) and her **attention** (past failures, perceived weakness, and fear of letting herself down).

She was arguing for her inability to become strong. If my grandfather were still alive, he'd have jumped right in with a cliché Maine-ism: "You just can't get there from here!"

That way of thinking won't get her where she's trying to go.

You can't create an identity of strength while you continue to view yourself through a filter of weakness.

I challenged her to resist coming at this desire from the perspective of the problem.

I asked her, "Is it possible for you? Is it possible for you to become that strong person you want to be?"

Instead of saying "Yes" or "No," she hedged. "Well, I mean...not the way things have been going—"

I cut her off. "Is it possible? Yes or no."

"Yes," she replied. "It is possible."

"Do you want it?"

"Yes."

"Is it important?"

"Yes, but you wouldn't know it by the way—"

I cut her off again. "You need to stop that. The past isn't relevant. Stay in the solution. Stop looking backwards unless you want to go that way. You can't carry the past with you and simultaneously create something. You can't cling to the limitation and also wish to be freed from it."

You probably do this, too.

It's fear-based thinking.

You detach from possibility and attach to fear and doubt. You detach from the present and attach to the past. Sure, it's how we protect our ego against the possibility of failure, but it's also how we keep ourselves from creating success.

This friend of mine was taking her past experiences and projecting them onto her present. She was stepping out of her present potential and going back into the past. She was acting as if her past in some way limits her present and future. It doesn't, unless she continues to choose it.

You decide: **Do you believe more in your past or in your present and your potential?**

Will you cling to your fear or chase your growth?

Do your choices back that up? Your thoughts? Your emotions? Your focus?

Don't fall into the trap of telling yourself that the way things have been in the past is the way they are right now. You get to **decide** how things are right now—how *you* are right now. With every one of your choices, you make that decision.

My Masters Club friend had a really important decision to make. She had to make it in that moment and she's going to have to make it a thousand more times in the weeks and months that follow.

Before we explore that important decision, let's take a closer look at the word "decide." As a former Latin major, I'm an unapologetic word geek!

In many languages, the preposition "de" means off or from. "Cide" comes from the Latin "caedere" which means cut. "Decide" means to cut off or cut from. When you make a decision, you are cutting off an option.

The decision my friend had to make is one you'll have to make too. **She had to cut off the belief stemming from the past so that she could embrace beliefs representative of what she wanted.** She had to cut off the story of the past patterns in order to open herself up to the possibilities and potential in front of her. To create change and develop the strength she desires, she will have to choose to focus on the fact that it *is* possible and she *is* capable. She's going to have to choose to focus on how she can be strong right now, today, in this moment. She has to decide, and have that decision be reflected in her thoughts and attention, that she is in fact free from everything that has happened in the past.

The only thing that links her to her past patterns is her belief in them. The only way they have any strength or power is if she continues to invest in them.

The story of the past simply isn't relevant anymore.

"It will work if you forget all the reasons it won't."

—PAULO COEHLO

How can you apply that idea in your life? What will it look like?

As *you* create change, there are new narratives you're going to have to create and old ones you will have to cut off.

That's your decision. Will you continue to endorse this belief or will you cut it off because it's no longer relevant or reflective of where you want to go?

QUESTIONS TO ASK

- What slows you down or gets in your way?
- What can you release that is no longer serving you?
- What thoughts, habits, or choices do not contribute to your best, happiest, healthiest life?
- How can you choose differently today?
- What are some behaviors, thoughts, patterns, or habits that don't reflect the best version of you?
- In what ways do you fuel them with your thoughts, attention, or choices?
- How might you make today different?
- What limitations do you argue for?
- How?
- What else is true?
- What change can you make this week to make other parts of your life flow more easily?
- In what ways are you arguing for the past or the problem?
- What else is possible?

SIX

Stories That Sabotage

"Remove the veils so I might see what is really happening here and not be intoxicated by my stories and my fears."

—ELIZABETH LESSER

Whether you're aware of it or not, you are constantly telling yourself stories—stories about who you are, how you act, and your patterns, abilities, and limitations.

You tell stories about what you're capable of, what your future looks like, what you're good at, bad at, and everything in-between. You manufacture stories about the people in your life, their intentions, and their feelings. I do it, too.

These stories box you in to a familiar experience and a limited scope of behavior. You're giving yourself a very small set of potential choices—those you've pulled from your past experiences.

You limit yourself to the problem and the past patterns. You confine yourself with walls you've built. These walls are made of beliefs you cling to about your weaknesses and limitations.

Remember that Rumi quote that changed my life? "Why do you stay in prison when the door is so wide open?"

Stories are simply patterns and problems you believe in. They can come from our past choices, fears, insecurities, or assumptions.

Here are some common stories or ways we define and describe ourselves—stories we tell ourselves and others that establish barriers to change.

I'm an emotional eater.

I have no self-control.

I'm bad with money.

I'm the fat one.

I'm inconsistent.

I'm a serial starter but never finish.

I get bored easily.

I'm not motivated.

Your thoughts and words about these stories make them stronger. **You are rehearsing the pattern when you think these thoughts.** When you repeat these statements to others, you're reminding yourself and boxing yourself in. You further reinforce and strengthen these stories with your choices. Each time you make a choice that is aligned with that story, the story gets stronger as you consciously (and subconsciously) believe in it even more.

You either maintain your present reality, replay your past, or create a change based on the way you think. **Your inner dialogue creates your entire experience of life.**

When you change your thoughts, you change your life.

I will never forget the exact moment I realized the damage my story was creating in my life. My story had been there for so long that I didn't even **recognize** it was a chosen set of beliefs that I was free to change. I didn't initially see these beliefs as a problem because they were the only way I had ever thought about myself and my choices. I had never considered that there might be a different way to think! I didn't realize that I had been confining myself with walls I was building each time I thought or shared this story. In hindsight, I can honestly say that my attachment to and emotional investment in this story was the primary thing keeping me from creating change in my life.

But there was a big problem I'd have to overcome in order to rewrite the story: I *believed* in my sad story. I believed my negative opinions of myself and I believed in the power of my past patterns of behavior. I didn't know *how* to believe something else.

I was in my late twenties when I first realized just how destructive my story was. I was doing well in my career. I had been promoted a couple times within a short period of time. I knew I was good at my job. I was routinely the first in my department to arrive at work and the last to leave. I never hesitated to work nights and weekends. I solved problems and worked hard.

I was newly married. My husband also had a great job. We bought a brand new home and adopted an adorable German shepherd puppy named Oakley. Despite "having it all," I was deeply unhappy with myself.

I weighed over 350 pounds and my weight was the biggest, most frustrating problem in my life. My husband wanted to start a family but I couldn't imagine carrying a baby *and* all the extra weight I couldn't seem to lose.

I had been unsuccessfully dieting since I was a kid and I didn't understand how I could be so focused, disciplined, and hardworking in my job but not with my weight. I certainly cared infinitely more about losing weight than I did about being good at my job. I wanted to be fit, lean, healthy, strong, and confident more than I wanted anything else, but it was *my own choices* that were holding me back.

I believed I just wasn't motivated and disciplined enough. I was convinced it would always be a struggle.

But I *was* motivated and disciplined. Not only was I thriving in my career, I had just paid off over $130,000 in debt in under two years through *intense* discipline and focus. It required *daily* motivation and I made it happen. There were obstacles and opportunities for excuses every day, but I overcame them and never quit.

I vividly remember driving home from work one day and wondering how I could be so motivated and disciplined with my career and my finances but fail so miserably with my pursuit of weight loss and my food choices.

How could I continue to blame my weight on being unmotivated and undisciplined when I was clearly capable of being highly motivated and disciplined in other areas of my life?

I started thinking about my perspectives on each of these areas of my life—my work, money, weight—and quickly saw the problem.

My story.

I *believed* I was great at my job. I *knew* I was a hard worker. I prided myself on learning new things, showing up early, staying late, and putting in the time and effort to be really good.

The same was true with my finances. The way I talked about getting out of debt was very clear: "I am getting out of debt. I don't care what we have to give up. This is important. I will make the sacrifices. Getting out of debt is worth more than frivolous spending."

There's a critical piece of my history that you need to understand: I hadn't always been a hard worker and I hadn't always been good with money. In my first job out of college, I was a pretty awful employee. I didn't show any initiative. I was lazy, unfocused, and lacked motivation. I did the minimum amount of work required to avoid getting fired. I'd go home on my lunch break and take a two-hour nap. I wasn't good with money. When I graduated college, the first thing I did was get a car loan and a credit card. When I got reimbursed from my first employer for some of my graduate school loans, I used the money to buy new furniture.

What would have happened if my professional story continued to be that I was lazy and unmotivated? What if I continued to tell myself I was too tired to get to the office early or too stressed to work on projects over the weekend? Would my professional reality have changed? Not a chance.

What would have happened if my story about money continued to be that I'd never get out of debt so there was no point in trying? What if I continued to tell myself that I wasn't disciplined enough to stick to a budget? Would my financial reality have changed so dramatically? Not a chance.

Those stories would have talked me out of action, motivation, and discipline. I would have talked myself into excuses, exceptions, doubt, and delay.

Because I was willing to change my story, I was able to change my life.

My *beliefs* about the areas of my life where I was thriving were the primary reason I did well. I decided that I could be a hard worker. It didn't matter that I hadn't been one before, I just knew it was possible. I *decided* to get good at my job. I put in the time and worked harder than people around me. I communicated clearly and I asked a lot of questions. When I didn't know something, I'd find answers. I volunteered for projects—I pursued hard work. I stopped placing blame and making excuses. I focused more on the solutions than the problems. I made the same change with my finances. I *decided* to change. I decided to give more to the goal than to the limitations.

Professionally and financially, I created a change one choice at a time.

Meanwhile, my story about food and my weight remained *unchanged*. I'm just the fat girl. I turn to food in response to stress. I'm great at losing weight and terrible at keeping it off. I'm an emotional eater. I'll never be consistent for long enough for it to make a difference. There's too far to go. It's too hard. Who cares? I'll start tomorrow.

My story about my weight was talking me *out* of action, motivation, and discipline, while my stories about my job and my finances were talking me *into* action, motivation, and discipline.

The issues with my weight weren't about my ability to be motivated or disciplined, but rather *my beliefs* about my ability to be motivated and disciplined.

All stories are descriptive. They are also *prescriptive*. Your story prescribes your future choices by defining and limiting your beliefs.

Your results reflect your story.

I was convincing myself that I couldn't lose weight. I had done a brilliant job at convincing myself of it.

What happens if you convince yourself of something every day, multiple times a day, for decades? You certainly won't exceed your own expectations.

I've heard it said that if you *don't* believe that your stories and beliefs matter, write "You suck, stupid!" on your child's bathroom mirror every single morning for ten years. Say it to them as they hop out of your car on the way to school each day. (But please, don't do that.)

Why *wouldn't* we do that? Because we understand the impact of our words on others. It's time to wake to the impact our own words—spoken and thought—have on us. It's major.

You will act in accordance with *your* story.

When you try to change your behavior without changing your story, you're asking for struggle, frustration, emotion, and inconsistency. You're asking for doubt. You're asking for excuses.

If you want to change your behavior, begin by changing your story. Just like you've created and reinforced the story about the problem, you are 100 percent capable, right now, of creating and supporting a story that reflects what you want and where you're going. You are 100 percent capable, right now, of letting go of the story about where you've been and what you don't want.

I had to change my personal story. But how? Like I told you, I *believed* all those things! I *didn't* believe that I was fit and lean and disciplined. I certainly wasn't going to tell myself a story that was categorically false.

And you shouldn't either.

If you know you're lying to yourself, you aren't fooling your brain. That won't work. **Your new story has to be one you believe in, but also one that reflects the positive change you want to create.**

I began very simply by redirecting all those negative thoughts to *I am capable of making great choices just for today.*

Yes, negativity and thoughts like, *I'm huge! I'm gross! I*

always go back to my old habits popped up all the time. But I am in control of whether or not I choose to stay with those thoughts and fuel them with my attention. So are you.

Every time I noticed those negative beliefs and unproductive stories was a chance to redirect them. **I am the thinker; I am not my thoughts.** I have the power to think something else. So do you.

I don't have to surrender to those thoughts. I don't have to stay with them or continue to agree with them. I simply have to redirect them.

I am capable of making great choices just for today.

I'd routinely get down on myself and start thinking about how far I had to go and how long it would take. I'd get frustrated that I had failed so many times before. Often, that story would loop in my mind almost unconsciously. But at some point, I *would* notice it. And when I did, I'd redirect it.

I am capable of making great choices just for today. What's my next great choice?

Sure, it would have been great to change my story to something more positive or empowering, like "I'm fit! I'm lean! I take impeccable care of myself!" But, quite frankly, that was beyond my level of belief at the time. It wasn't true for me yet.

I had to choose to focus on what I *could* believe. You do, too.

To be completely honest, there were some days I didn't feel capable of making good choices for one entire day. That felt like too much. On those days, I'd just make the new story even more simple and manageable:

I have one more good choice in me. I have one great hour in me. I am capable of making my next choice a great choice. What is one good choice I'm able and willing to make right now?

With consistent practice and repeated redirection, my story began to change, my level of belief increased and my results reflected the change.

Changing my story changed my life.

I do this work with my clients (and myself) every single day. We don't begin by changing their habits; we begin by improving their stories, because habits stem from stories. One of my clients would constantly tell me about how she had grown up in a family where everything centered around overeating and drinking in excess. She had long since moved out of her family home, but this continued to be the story she told herself and everyone close to her about food and alcohol.

One day I asked her, "Why do you keep leading with that story? Why do you keep telling yourself about the past? Why do you limit yourself with something that doesn't reflect what you want?" I already knew her family background, but she continued to remind me. Why was she making this a part of every conversation about change?

"Because it's who I am!" she told me.

Is it? Is it who you are or is it simply what you practiced in the past?

What you've experienced isn't who you are. It's not even what you *do* unless you choose to keep it alive through your practice. Your history isn't your identity. It's not your destiny. You don't have to continue to live these stories and submit to past patterns. You are free to let them go. And, if you want to move beyond the pattern, you *must* let it go!

While these regurgitations of history often satisfy our egos and justify our present patterns or lack of progress, they certainly don't move us forward. They hold us back.

Are there stories about your past you continue to revisit in your thoughts and words? What are the stories you cling to that justify or validate the behaviors you want to move beyond?

What if you stopped telling that story? What if you decided there was another way to be and gave your energy to the new story?

Growing up, we celebrated everything with food. Lots of food. Though there was always tension between my mom and me over my weight, our family as a whole loved to make food the center of celebrations.

In fact, we've had a holiday mantra for decades: eat like a pig!

I'm 100 percent serious. Though I was the token fat person in my family, everyone would joke, "It's Christmas! Eat like a pig! It's Easter! Eat like a pig!" Over the years, it jokingly morphed into "It's the third Tuesday in June! Eat like a pig! It's raining out! Eat like a pig!"

That's a story from my past, nothing more, nothing less. It is not who I am. It's also not "how I was raised." It's merely something that happened. It doesn't limit how I'm able to act on holidays. It doesn't in any way remove or impair my ability to make choices on any day of the week or year.

Let's look at where you might benefit from changing your thoughts and your stories. Think about some of the beliefs you have about yourself. Consider the positive beliefs and also the negative ones.

What do you believe about areas where you struggle?

What do you believe about areas where you're thriving?

What's the difference?

What do you believe about your potential for change?

What do you believe about who you are and how you act as it relates to your goal? What stories are you holding onto that you can choose to leave in the past?

If your primary goal is to get out of debt, what do you believe about yourself and money? Earning potential? Spending? Discipline? Are you telling stories about people who have influenced you and their money habits? Can you see that you don't have to submit to those beliefs? How might you change your story?

If your primary goal is weight loss, what do you believe about yourself and your habits as they relate to food and weight loss? Are you telling stories about the past? Are you telling stories about other people's relationships with food? Are you telling stories about problems, limitations, frustrations, or barriers? Can you see that you don't have to submit to those beliefs? Are they helpful? Are they not helpful? Are they related to the problem or to the solution? Do they move you in the direction of the change you want or do they keep you attached to the behaviors that created the problem?

These are stories—patterns of belief that stand as pillars in your mind, supporting the patterns you currently have.

If you want to change your patterns, change your story. Change the thoughts you have and the words you speak.

Your thoughts are instructions to your brain.

Nearly every day, I get emails from listeners or clients that say something along the lines of:

"I need help. I don't know what to do. I really need to lose weight but I have no self-control. I make these plans and I set all these grand intentions, but then I don't follow through. I can do it for a couple days, but I always go back to my old habits. I seriously don't know what's wrong with me. I just can't stay motivated."

My response is the same each time:

"Dear listener—the first thing I want you to do is go back and reread your email to me as if it were a set of instructions to your brain, because it is. Are those the instructions you want to give your brain on how to think, choose, and behave? Your words are both descriptive and prescriptive. You are prescribing to yourself a pattern of behavior. You're taking the past and projecting it onto the present. Knowing that, how might you think about this differently?"

Their story is jumping off the page: *I have no self-control. I don't follow through. I always go back to my old habits. I can't stay motivated.*

Okay. I believe you. Your results reflect your story.

These are all limiting beliefs you are choosing to tell yourself. You are *selling* them to yourself and convincing yourself that you don't have power.

You're minimizing yourself—making your past greater than your potential.

Approximately 90 percent of your choices are made on the subconscious level, and your subconscious acts in the way you instruct it to act. Your thoughts, words, and actions are instructions to your brain.

Think about all the times you've said, "I have no patience

in traffic." That's a belief you are selling yourself, a story you are telling yourself. Of course you're *more* than capable of being not only patient in traffic, but also of being grateful to be safely nestled in your car. But, you've convinced yourself otherwise with your story.

If you tell your subconscious that you can be great for a few days, but then always blow it, **you've given it both instruction and permission to give up after a few days.**

"Be careful of the words you speak—they become the house you live in!"

—HAFIZ

That quote hangs in my kitchen to remind me of the power of stories. Thoughts become things.

Indulge me for a second and imagine you're driving down a dirt road. You drive this road every day. Over time and with repetition, your tires will form grooves in the dirt, right?

The more frequently you travel that same path, the deeper the grooves will be. Eventually, grooves become ruts.

The deeper the rut, the harder it becomes to drive outside of them. Your car wants to travel along that pre-formed, well-practiced path.

This is also true with your stories and choices. The story, repeated, creates a well-worn path that your choices travel down. Your choices want to align with those tracks of repetition, and the more you engage in the story, the deeper the grooves become.

No matter what your story is, don't hold so tight. You don't need to keep returning to the story.

Don't cling to the circumstances or rationalizations.

Be open to the idea that there might be another perspective you've been missing. Be open to another version of your reality. Your familiar version of the truth isn't the *only* version of the truth. Be open to the notion that you don't have to keep revisiting the past.

This way of challenging your thoughts can also be applied to ways you think about work and personal relationships. I mentioned earlier that I personally practice this daily. Recently, I realized I had a story about being a business owner that wasn't working for me at all. It was creating stress and struggle.

I recognized the story because I was feeling overwhelmed and constantly rushed in my work. I took a step back to ask, "What are my thoughts about my work that are contributing to these feelings?" Remember: our feelings are almost always driven by our thoughts. If you feel overwhelmed, there's a thought process generating that feeling. When you change your thoughts, you change your feelings.

When I wrote down my thoughts about work, I fully understood why I felt so out of control and recognized the need for a new story.

At the time, my story about work was, *I'm swamped! I am never caught up. The list keeps growing and I can't get ahead. I'm rushing from one project to the next, one fire to another, and I always have something else I need to be doing. It's unceasing. I can't rest. I can't stop. I'm exhausted.*

All those thoughts felt both real and true, so I started asking myself questions because I know that my truth isn't the only truth.

Is that the only way to view my work?

What else might be true?

Does it have to be this way?

How do I feel when I believe those thoughts?

Where might I be wrong?

What other perspectives are available to me?

To even get to the point where you're willing to answer these questions, you have to be willing to set aside your ego and value *getting it right* over *being right*. You don't *have* to adopt a new set of beliefs, but at least be willing to explore them.

Here's what I realized about my work:

I *could* do less. No one makes me put out three podcasts each week or daily blogs. *I* created the expectation that I'd respond to every email; no one requires that of me. I set that standard. I could absolutely make changes to be less busy, scale back my obligations, or hire help. I could slow down. I choose to rush. No one makes me rush.

My problem wasn't the business, it was my thoughts about it. My new story centered around the fact that *I* set the standards for work, and if I don't like them, I'm free to change them. I'm not a victim of standards I've set. Why stay in prison when the door is so wide open?

That line of thinking, questioning, and honesty led me to reduce the number of podcasts and blogs I put out each week and not take new clients over the summer.

I wouldn't have made those changes with the original

story that had me as the victim at the center. But I'm *not* a victim. *I am the solution.* I have more control than I often choose to realize or act on. So do you.

Divorce the story of the past so you can step into your full potential here in the present.

QUESTIONS TO ASK

- What are some of the stories you have about yourself, your circumstances, or your past that aren't serving you?
- What might be *more* true than the story you've been telling yourself?
- How might you change your perspective?
- What are you not seeing when you tell this story or describe things this way?
- What other perspectives are there?

SEVEN

Start with Your Thoughts

"You must learn a new way to think before you can master a new way to be."

—MARIANNE WILLIAMSON

When it comes to creating personal change, there are a million possible levers to pull. There are countless changes you *could* make and, at some point, you've probably considered most of them. You could focus on losing weight, paying down debt, watching less television, getting more sleep, or spending more time with your family. The list is nearly endless.

This is where many of us get lost. There are so many options that we either become paralyzed by indecision or constantly jump from one change to another, never establishing consistency or identifying what *really* works. Without consistency, change requires a lot of effort but doesn't deliver significant results. This is what leads to spinning your wheels.

It's important to realize that all the possible starting points—all the possible action steps you *could* take—are *not* created equal. To make change easier and more likely to stick, you have to pick the *right* change to make.

In their book, *The 4 Disciplines of Execution*, authors Chris McChesney and Sean Covey help problem solvers figure out *where* to focus their efforts by differentiating between lead and lag measures.

Lag measures are your outcomes: weight loss, less debt, more money in savings, or running a six-minute mile. In the context of business, a lag measure might include hitting a revenue target or sales quota. **Lag measures are the endpoint you're working toward.** When pursuing goals, most people focus their efforts on those endpoints.

The authors make a case for why focusing on lag measures, or endpoints, is a *mistake*. Instead, they explain why you should focus on *lead* measures. **Lead measures are the actions that predict and influence the endpoint.** If the lag measure (endpoint) is weight loss, lead measures might include journaling, eating more vegetables, reducing processed foods, following The Golden Rules of Carbs and Fat Loss, or creating new beliefs and perspectives around food. Lead measures are factors that are completely within your control that predict and influence your end goal.

You have far *less* control over the endpoint than you do the factors that influence it.

Let's consider an example. A real estate agent might set a goal to sell more homes. Selling more homes is a **lag measure**; it's an endpoint.

Lead measures, actions, and behaviors that both predict and influence the goal might include things like calling more prospective clients, showing more homes to each buyer, or reaching out to people who have listed their home for sale by owner.

When an agent aggressively focuses on the lead measures, which predict and influence their end goal, they create more progress than if they broadly focus on trying to sell more homes.

For almost every goal, because you cannot *directly* influence the outcome, your energy should be invested in the attitudes and behaviors that predict and influence the end goal you're trying to reach.

If your goal is weight loss, the only thing you directly control are the choices and behaviors that predict and influence weight loss, like what you eat, how much you eat, and eliminating the excuses that get in the way.

For every goal, identify the lead measures that influence and predict the lag measure. Then, give your energy to those things. It's the *efficient* way to create change we're trying to pursue.

What behaviors both predict and influence the goal you want to achieve?

Once you have those things in mind, there's one more critical piece of information:

Not all the factors that predict and influence your goal are created equal. Some will have a dramatic impact. Some won't have much impact at all. I'm going to help you simplify this process.

There is one lead measure that will produce the most dramatic result. It's the starting point that will keep you off the hard road where you spin your wheels, expending effort without return.

The ultimate lead measure is **your thoughts.**

Optimizing your thoughts—how and what you think—is the lead measure with the highest return on investment.

You might think this sounds woo-woo and hippy-dippy, but it's not. This is **not** a puffy cloud and marshmallow touchy-feely strategy. It is both practical and effective because **your thoughts drive your choices.**

I told you that to create change you'd need to check your ego, remember? Be open to this idea. It *will* make change easier.

Think about it for a second. You've finished dinner. You aren't hungry but you just *want* something. Ever been there?

You think, *I just want a little something. Dark chocolate with a spoonful of almond butter is totally better than cookies or ice cream. And, I mean, it's so small, is it really gonna make a difference? Plus, I've been pretty good all day. I'll just finish off those dark chocolate squares. In fact, eating them tonight just means they won't be here to tempt me tomorrow!*

Via your thoughts, you've talked yourself into dessert. You've effectively convinced yourself. You made a case for it; you negotiated for it and came to the decision by way of your thoughts.

Your thoughts drive your choices.

Different thoughts in the same situation can lead to a completely different choice. Consider this alternate way of thinking. You aren't hungry after dinner but you just want a little something. You think, *Oooh, that dark chocolate would be so good. But you know, I'm not hungry. Food always tastes better when I'm hungry, and I'm sure that moment will come soon. I'll wait until then. Or, just for today, no dessert. I just ate. My body doesn't need fuel right now.*

It doesn't take willpower and discipline. When you choose to think differently, you act differently. Remember: white knuckles are red flags. Make change easier by **optimizing and altering the thoughts that influence and predict your choices**.

Different thoughts generate different choices. **It always works that way.** Your thoughts will talk you into or out of every choice you make. Your thoughts are the lead measure that has the greatest impact on the change you want to create.

You are the thinker. You can change your thoughts at any moment, and changing your thoughts is one of the most effective ways to change your actions.

Too often we look at *choices* as independent factors we can attack directly. We try to use white-knuckle willpower to change our choices, but **if you fail to change your thoughts, you continue to struggle.**

For as long as there is a lack of alignment between your thoughts and the choices you want to make, there will be inconsistency and struggle.

Every choice is made based on the series of thoughts that precede it.

Let's look at another example.

You're trying to eat clean but talk yourself into one of the homemade brownies in the break room. After you've enjoyed it, you choose a guilt response and think, *Well, I blew it! What's the point in eating clean for the rest of the day? I might as well get these cravings out of my system so I can be super strict tomorrow!*

A single brownie turns into a full-blown binge, not because you don't have control, but because you used the thing over which you have the *most* control, your thoughts, to make a case for the binge. Every slip becomes a slide, and it all started with a thought you chose about the choice you made. You created the meaning, by way of your thoughts, and that drove your choice.

Here's how thoughts and choices occur, and how they form habits and beliefs.

Your thoughts drive your choices.

Your choices, repeated, form your habits.

Your habits create your results.

Your results inform your beliefs.

Your beliefs then generate more of the same thoughts that justify the same choices that produce the same results.

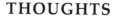

BELIEF   **THOUGHTS**

RESULTS   **CHOICES**

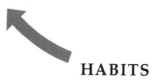

HABITS

This can be an amazingly powerful and transformative cycle, once understood and optimized, or it can feel like a death trap, preventing all desired progress and making you feel like your habits control you.

But your habits don't control you because you can change your thoughts, and that will open you up to improved choices.

This is the starting point for all change. You change the entire cycle when you change your thoughts.

If you look at each of these stops on the wheel of change as a potential starting point, you'll quickly see why starting with thoughts is most effective.

Let's look at what happens with the most common approach to change, which instructs you to focus exclusively on adopting different behaviors. "Just eat less," they say.

Undoubtedly, you're initially on board. You know what to do and how to do it. But, for some reason, you're not doing the work. Instead, you're giving in to excuses and creating exceptions, all the while wondering why you're sabotaging yourself.

The habit of excuse and exception is created. You aren't

getting results. Your lack of results and recurring disappointment reinforce the belief that you can't change and don't have what it takes. You start thinking, *What's the point? Why do I bother? What's wrong with me?* What choices do those thoughts drive? More of the same: the choices that created the problem in the first place. Sounds a lot like the hard road, right? Like the white-knuckle willpower approach.

Choice begins with thought. If you want to change your choices and actions, start with your thoughts. It will be far more effective.

If you think of eating healthy as a chore and a burden, you're going to grab ahold of any and every excuse to indulge. If, on the other hand, you consistently change your thoughts about eating healthy, reminding yourself of how great it makes you feel and how much worse you feel when you overindulge, your food choices become far easier. If you think about how far you have to go until you reach your goal, you'll feel discouraged, not motivated. But when you think about how you totally have one good choice in you, that choice instantly feels easier.

One of the most insidious barriers to change I encounter with my clients is the one that most people feel best about: **great intentions.**

Great intentions show up as assurances that you will do better tomorrow or start fresh on Monday.

No matter how focused you are on improving your choices, if your thoughts still reflect your promises to start tomorrow or do better tomorrow, you won't create the change you crave. You'll continue dismissing the opportunity.

Changing your thoughts changes the entire game.

When you decide to change your thoughts from *I'll do better tomorrow* to *I will win this day*, you change your entire operating system.

In a moment, as you redirect to a new way of thinking, you reject the thought that justifies the choice you want to avoid. **When your thoughts reflect the way you want to be, you'll make a choice that creates the change you desire.** You'll build a habit of doing what you can *now* instead of making a case for *later*. That shift will drive results. It will foster belief in your ability to create change and in your ability to be different than you've been.

You'll establish a habit of focusing on what you can do now, instead of what you can put off until later. That powerful change begins with your thoughts.

No matter how badly you want to exercise more, if your

thoughts remain focused on how you hate to work out, don't have the time or energy, or how you'll start tomorrow, you probably won't be working out consistently anytime soon.

Discipline and willpower force change in *the things you do*. Discipline and willpower don't change who you are and how you think. When you change how you think, your choices will naturally improve with dramatically less effort. It won't matter if you had a bad day or you're traveling or on vacation, your new thoughts will drive new choices.

HOW? HOW DO YOU CHANGE YOUR THOUGHTS?

You might be thinking that it is difficult to change the way you think, but it's not. It is actually very simple. You're not alone if you're thinking that you usually don't even *notice* your thoughts. Don't worry if you're wondering, *How do I pay more attention to my thoughts? I have great intentions, but when I'm in the swing of my day, I often react out of habit and unconsciously choose past patterns.* Most of us have a tendency to drift and not pay close attention to our thoughts or the choices they create. Life happens, and our focus on creating change gets overshadowed by our work, our habits, our families, and so much more.

Fortunately, you can begin to change your thoughts right

now, at this very moment. It doesn't hinge on your ability to catch yourself before reaching into the box of Goldfish crackers.

You'll begin optimizing *any* thought at absolutely any time! You'll start by changing your thoughts in any moment you *are* paying attention.

For example, instead of thinking about why you can't change your choices and what's in the way of that change, think about why and how you *can*.

Thinking differently is a skill built through practice, and the practice is much broader than just thinking differently about your choices related to your goals. For example, as I write this, I'm sitting in a Starbucks. A few minutes ago, I was feeling a little irritated by how loud it is in here. A few kids are yelling, a man is talking loudly on his cell phone, and there's employee training going on behind the counter. Why was I feeling irritated? It's not the people and the noise that irritate me; it's my thoughts about them. Here's how I know:

Instead of thinking, *Ugh! Be quiet! No one wants to hear your conversation. I can't concentrate!* I simply choose a different perspective. *I chose to work from here. If it's too loud, I can leave. I can go home. I can go to the library. I can sit outside. This isn't my private office, it's a public coffee shop. If I wanted silence, I came to the wrong place.*

This, and every moment, is an opportunity to practice the skill of thinking differently.

Changing the way I think doesn't mean I have to convince myself that I love the noise. It simply means I can choose to think about it differently.

When you notice any negative emotion, you have an immediate opportunity to practice the superpower of changing your thoughts. Whether the negativity is in response to work stress, a snarky email, or how your jeans fit, you can change your perspective and think about it differently.

For example, I practice thinking differently every day when I'm getting ready to go to the gym.

I have a habit of thinking, *I don't want to go. I'm tired. I don't want to sweat. I have so much work to do. I don't have time.* When I recognize that "ugh" feeling, it reminds me to change my perspective. There's always a different perspective I can choose.

I love how I feel after a workout. I don't want to take this body and its ability to move for granted. Someday I may wish I could work out. Today I can, so today I will. I'll be glad I did. Get going, kiddo. Up and at 'em.

This is something you can also practice in hindsight. After you've made a choice, ask yourself, **what was I thinking when I made that choice?**

Though the choice has already been made, the practice of asking and answering that question will increase your awareness of how your thoughts were impacting your choices. Building awareness, even if initially practiced in hindsight, increases *overall* awareness.

Changing your thoughts ultimately requires that you pay more attention. To participate in the solution, you have to increase your participation in the present moment.

The truth is, because we go through so many of our days on autopilot, rarely functioning as more than a reactive passenger in our own lives, we haven't practiced this innate superpower we all possess.

Choosing your thoughts is a daily practice—often an hourly practice—that will make this work of creating a new story infinitely easier. The more you practice, the easier it becomes.

You are not a victim of the thoughts in your head. Do

not convince yourself that you have no control over negativity or excuses. It's simply not true.

You can always redirect your attention. You are the thinker. You are not your thoughts.

Years ago, someone asked me about the best advice I ever received. Without a doubt it was, **learn to stop listening to yourself and start talking to yourself.** Or, as author and designer Debbie Millman was instructed by a sage fortune cookie, "Avoid compulsively making things worse."

You don't *ever* have to follow a thought down a rabbit hole of anxiety or negativity. Recognize when the thoughts you're thinking aren't serving you. In those moments, change them!

Most of the thoughts we have are at best not productive, and at worst having a negative impact on our mood and achievement.

Remember our conversation about spinning your wheels. Are your thoughts helping you create a solution? Are they even related to the solution? Are your thoughts productive? Are they destructive?

Think about the last time you were in line at the grocery

store and the person in front of you not only had a million coupons, they also needed a price check. Maybe they had eighteen items in the ten items or fewer lane. If you're at all like me, you might have felt irritated and impatient. You might have stood there wondering if you should switch lines and thinking less-than-kind thoughts about the shopper in front of you.

I've noticed this kind of first-world frustration when I'm getting off an airplane. I'm standing there, ready go, able to grab my stuff and file off in an orderly fashion, but it seems some people aren't on the same page. As I stand there waiting, I'm glad my thoughts aren't being broadcast over the intercom: *Seriously? What is so complicated about getting off a plane? Grab your stuff; move your feet. Let's go, guys.*

It's not the situation that annoys me; my thoughts about the situation lead to feeling annoyed.

In those moments, I remind myself that I can think differently about any situation. If I think about it differently, I'll feel better, so I use the situation to intentionally flex my thought-control muscle. The more I practice changing my thoughts, the more capable I am to optimize my thoughts in *all* moments. I'm building the habit of choosing thoughts that serve me in every situation, while rejecting thoughts that don't serve me.

Build the skill when you can so you have it when you need it.

I don't *have* to think about the line at the grocery store in a negative way. I don't have to think of the slow deplaning process as an inconvenience. Those perspectives are a *choice*, even if a practiced one, and I am always free to choose different thoughts.

When I'm getting irritated about traffic, I redirect my thoughts to simple gratitude that I'm safe in my car. Often, traffic accumulates because someone isn't so fortunate. I think about the day my dad died in a car accident. I'm sure traffic backed up around the scene and I hate to think that someone was annoyed by the inconvenience of having to wait while first responders rushed to his side or while they removed his body. I want to be someone who has more respect for others than what I show when I get irritated by the inconvenience of waiting. Sure, sometimes the traffic is because of construction or something unrelated to an accident. In those moments, I still choose gratitude for my safety. I still choose to practice patience.

When the deplaning process is making my blood pressure rise (more accurately, when my *thoughts* about the deplaning process are making my blood pressure rise), I'll instead think about how great it is that we landed safely and how blessed I am to have the luxury of plane travel.

I remind myself how fortunate I am to be able to gather my luggage quickly. Some people can't do it themselves. I refuse to turn my blessings into burdens. Or maybe this delay is simply happening because I need a reminder to calm down and be patient.

There's a great fringe benefit to changing your thoughts—you'll automatically improve your mood. Life is short. Don't be such a grump.

THE PRACTICE OF OPTIMIZING YOUR THOUGHTS

"If you believe you aren't good enough, think of how many chances you'll have in a week to prove it to yourself."

—BONNIE KELLY

There are three different ways you can practice this (and we all need to practice as much as we can). I'm not suggesting you stand in line and tell yourself you love waiting. No lying. No sarcasm.

I didn't convince myself I love the noisy Starbucks environment; I reminded myself how many other options I have. I didn't tell myself I love waiting to get off the plane; I reminded myself how lucky I am to be safe and able to gather my own belongings without assistance. **When I was at my heaviest, I didn't tell myself I loved my body; I told myself I am capable of changing it.** I didn't tell myself that I always make awesome choices; I told myself that I always have one good choice in me.

Let's explore the three different kinds of redirects you can practice.

- The neutral redirect
- The empowering redirect
- The positive redirect

The neutral redirect turns your attention away from the negative thought and toward a different topic.

The empowering redirect shifts your attention from what is wrong or what you *can't* do toward something within your control.

The positive redirect turns your attention toward a positive belief about yourself or your circumstance.

We can see how these would work in the grocery store example. The next time you feel frustrated by the grocery store line, consider these options:

The neutral redirect: Use your wait time to check Instagram or catch up on email.

The empowering redirect: You can get in a different line

if you'd like. You can leave your items in the store and head home without them. No one is forcing you to stand in this line.

The positive redirect: Here you are, able to buy groceries for yourself, able to shop on your own, able to prepare a great meal. Refuse to turn your blessings into burdens.

Let's do some practice with these three redirects on an example that is more closely associated with a goal you want to achieve.

Let's say you find your thoughts revolving around the fact that **you have no self-control**. You're beating yourself up for breaking a promise you made to yourself and you're feeling like you just can't change. It's not possible. No matter how good your intentions are, you cave to temptation every time.

As soon as you notice the thoughts (even if it's after the fact), redirect your attention to a neutral, empowering, or positive thought.

From: I have no self-control.

To neutral: What's on Netflix that I'm excited to watch?

Empowering: I have total control. There's a difference

between not having control and not taking control. I'm the one making the choices. I simply need more practice.

Positive: Here I am, aware of what I don't want and desiring change! That's a critical first step! What's my next best choice?

The neutral redirect might seem like a total waste of time, but it's not. You might not be in the mood for an empowering or positive redirect, but at least you're no longer giving your energy to the thoughts associated with the problem. Sure, you'll benefit *more* from giving your energy to the solution, but any neutral thought, including thoughts about the color of your socks, is better than thoughts that fuel the problem.

For the sake of clarity, a neutral redirect is *not* a negative redirect. You don't want to switch your attention from thinking you have no self-control to thinking about how you hate your job or your arms are too fat. You aren't shifting your energy to something negative; you're intentionally changing your focus and attention and putting it on something that is neutral.

The more you practice these redirects in any situation, the easier it becomes in *every* situation. The more deeply rooted your belief in the problem, the more opportunities you will have to practice, and therefore the faster you can improve. Said another way, the more often you find yourself thinking about the problem, the more opportunities exist for you to practice these redirects. The more you practice, the faster you create change.

I'll be really clear about the hardest part: **you have to be willing to let go of the problem and not cling to it simply because it's familiar or makes you feel justified in your lack of progress. You don't have to retreat into the familiar story of the problem.**

I worked for months with a client whose story was that she is an emotional eater. She was struggling to change this pattern of behavior, in large part because she identified more with the problem than with the solution. More of her thoughts, words, and choices supported the problem (emotional eating) than the solution or change she wanted to create. To help her establish a new way of thinking about it, we started with a question. As we'll talk more about in the coming chapters, questions are a powerful tool to help you create new ways of thinking.

After she made a solid case for her emotional eating, including how long she's been doing it, why she does it, and a summary of her past failed attempts to change, I asked her a question.

What *else* is true about your emotional eating?

Here are some of the things she told me.

It doesn't make me feel better.

When I choose it, not only do I feel awful, but I've missed a chance to practice creating a new pattern of behavior.

No one is forcing me to be an emotional eater.

It is possible for me to not eat when I'm emotional; I just need more practice. There's nothing about me or food that makes that impossible.

I've been choosing what feels easiest even though there are lots of different options.

I can do hard things.

Emotional eating is a past pattern unless I choose it right now.

Practicing the three redirects was the stepping-stone to her new story. When she felt drawn to eat in response to emotion or when she was thinking about this pattern of behavior, she'd practice one of these three.

Neutral redirect: Enough of that. I need to work on this presentation for my meeting tomorrow.

Empowering redirect: I am in control of my choices. I can choose differently in this moment. Since transformation is now, this is a chance to practice.

Positive redirect: I am completely capable of making myself feel better, if I decide to. What choices can I make right now that will help me feel better?

IT'S NOT RELEVANT

"He suffers more than necessary, who suffers before it is necessary."

—SENECA

Imagine for a minute that it's mid-winter and the temperatures outside are far below freezing. You've cranked the heat inside, but it's still super drafty. You don't understand why it's not warming up until you realize that someone left three windows open upstairs! All your heat is pouring out the windows and the cold air is being invited in! You slam the windows shut. The house can't warm up with all the heat escaping.

If you are struggling to create change in your life and changing your behavior feels hard, there is likely a lot of motivation, energy, and focus escaping, just like the heat out the open window. You have enough motivation, energy, and focus; you just can't continue wasting it.

This, too, stems back to your thoughts.

If you think you don't have enough motivation, time, or effort to create that change you want in your life, I'll bet that part of the reason for that sense of "not enough" stems from the wasted time and energy going into **factors that simply aren't relevant.**

When you nip that inefficiency and unintended loss in the bud, change becomes easier. The hard road starts looking much more like easy street. Improving your ability to recognize when your thoughts simply are not relevant will free up all sorts of energy and emotion that you can use to create a change.

One of my clients shared with me that she wants to create the same improvements with food that she has already worked hard to make with alcohol. She used to be a binge drinker. Her first couple days without alcohol were hard, and she was absolutely miserable. But once she got to the third or fourth day without it, she remembered just how great she feels when she's *not* drinking. The contrast she created by avoiding alcohol completely for a few days helped her completely reframe her thoughts about drinking. Instead of being caught in the allure of alcohol, she was more drawn to how great she felt *without* it. She couldn't experience that contrast without first giving herself the experience of change and pushing through the initial hard days. She cut herself off from the belief that not drinking meant missing out. She chose a new belief, fueled by practice, that she misses out on far *more* when she *does* drink.

Having created that experience with alcohol, she wanted to do the same thing with food. She had a pattern of binge eating and, as things were, the temptation to overeat was greater than the desire to eat healthy. She was much more practiced in turning to food than she was in *not* turning to food.

She and I were talking through how she could generate enough momentum to have a few great, controlled days with food to find out how good she could feel without binging. To create the contrast bias, she was going to have to resist temptation and work through the hard days of early change. To create the momentum for that effort, she'd have to change her thoughts.

While we brainstormed ways to reframe the way she thinks about food and binging, she randomly started talking about how she recently became really jealous of a friend after seeing a picture on social media. This friend had made different choices and seemed to be living a healthy, happy life. She shared that her friend was fit, lean, and successful in her career. After listening to her lament the path she wished she had taken, I stopped her.

"That's not relevant," I told her. "You're wasting energy comparing yourself to someone else and dwelling on past opportunities. You aren't focused on what you can do. You aren't focused on today. You're giving your energy away to someone else, the past, and what you didn't do."

Metaphorically, she was opening up all the windows, letting the heat escape.

Don't let comparison drain your energy.

Don't let the past drain your energy.

Don't let what you can't do drain your energy.

Identify which thoughts and stories aren't relevant. They are artificial constraints you're manufacturing. Leave them behind. Shut them down. Do not fuel them with your attention. You are the thinker. Use these moments to practice thinking differently by redirecting your thoughts.

The very next day, I was having a conversation with a middle-aged client who shared with me that she wants to stop overthinking. It's exhausting her, and this habit leaves her spinning her wheels with options and then doing nothing at all. Her overthinking makes every choice harder than it needs to be. She wastes mental energy, and time, in considering every possible option. The pattern isn't working for her.

We talked about creating the experience of just **one day** with less thinking and more doing. I asked if she was able to practice simple decision-making criteria (like "yes" or "no" instead of a two-hour debate) for just one day, and she was on board. We talked about breaking out of the thinking pattern and into the *doing* pattern by asking simple questions like "What choice brings me closer to my goal?" "Is this my best?" "Is it a hell yes? If not, it's a no."

Thinking less; doing more. Taking an easier road instead of staying on the harder one.

A few minutes into our conversation about the solution and what her practice will look like, she interjected and said, "It's weird. My kids are off to college and I'm just in this different phase of life, and it's an adjustment."

Her solution energy went out the window when she entertained that unrelated thought.

While her comments were true, they were simply not relevant. When you're locked in on a solution, don't allow yourself these tangents. Don't retreat into a story.

Don't misunderstand me. Some people will choose to

interpret this as me saying I don't care about my clients' circumstances. That couldn't be further from the truth. **What I'm trying to illuminate is your tendency to follow wild, winding rabbit trails of thoughts and ideas, which let your energy, motivation, and focus fly out the window, leaving you with not enough remaining to be a joyful change agent in your own life.**

The hard road is littered with tangents and ideas that aren't relevant to the change you want to create.

Continuing down that rabbit hole of thought, she'd have argued for the fact that life is hard, change is hard, and she's doing the best she can. While there's nothing inherently wrong with those thoughts, I wanted her, and you, to practice giving energy to the solution without inviting irrelevant distractions. I wanted her to recognize when she is distracting herself with thoughts, problems, and considerations that simply aren't relevant.

Does her kids moving out have anything to do with her practice of simple decision-making? Nope. Does it in any way alter what she can do today? Nope, it's just a narrative. It's an energy vacuum.

If you're giving your energy to a solution or trying to resolve a problem, give your energy to that. **Don't loop in**

parts of a different story that aren't related. They will only slow you down and steal your focus and momentum.

Ruthlessly ask yourself the following questions:

Is this relevant?

Is it related to me or someone else?

Is it related to what I can do now or am I dwelling in the past or the future?

Is this a necessary consideration in order for me to take action?

Is it part of the solution? Is it part of what I want and am trying to create?

ALL-OR-NOTHING THINKING

We can't talk about the power of your thoughts without addressing the malignant pattern of all-or-nothing thinking.

We can all relate to the fact that the all-or-nothing approach doesn't work in *any* pursuit. **In fact, I'd argue that all-or-nothing is another way of saying** *inconsistent*.

Many people will define themselves (confine themselves) by saying, "I'm totally all-or-nothing," as if it's the only way they can be. However, if we had them replace "all-or-nothing" with "inconsistent," the solution would immediately become more clear. All-or-nothing is a choice. There are other options.

An all-or-nothing inconsistent approach doesn't work when it comes to food, fitness, money, relationships, or career. We often know it doesn't work but choose it anyway. To create lasting success, you have to leave that approach behind.

Overcoming a pattern of all-or-nothing thinking requires just two things:

1. Self-awareness
2. Practice

That's it. It doesn't require white-knuckle willpower or any complicated plan or program. You can all overcome it with those two simple elements.

Self-awareness is required because all-or-nothing behaviors are nothing more than a perspective you talk yourself into. You convince yourself via flawed logic and a limited acknowledgment of the truth. You *know* that it's not effective to vacillate between all-in and all-out. Any negotiation in favor of it reflects incomplete thoughts. Self-awareness helps you notice that.

All-or-nothing patterns are fueled by your thoughts and executed in your choices.

Some of the most common ways we talk ourselves into it are with thoughts like *I'll indulge today and it'll be out of my system so I'll eat super clean tomorrow.*

I already screwed up, so I've already ruined the day.

What is implied in that logic is that change is a zero-sum game. You convince yourself that if you failed one choice, the entire day is lost.

The only thing that logic accomplishes is becoming a master beginner who never successfully finishes.

That won't work.

A client emailed me the other day explaining that she had a terrible weekend. She promised herself to eat clean but ended up having a couple drinks and some dessert.

From there, she said, things went downhill. She overate, overindulged, and felt absolutely terrible.

I asked her to share with me how she talked herself into the choices after the initial choice to drink. **This is the self-awareness piece.** What thoughts did you think to convince yourself to respond that way?

Here was her thought process: *Well, I already screwed up, so what's the point?*

That's the logic that makes a case for the all-or-nothing approach. It will never work.

Screw it. I blew it is a story. It's a grossly incomplete thought. It's dramatic and, more importantly, it's not effective.

We choose these half-baked dismissals because, in the moment, they are permissive. They give us permission to indulge, permission to do what feels good in the moment, and permission to put our goals on hold.

If you are telling yourself there is a problem, engage in solving it. If drinks and dessert are a problem, what is the solution? Practice thinking in complete thoughts.

It's not the brownie that's the problem. The brownie didn't create the all-or-nothing pattern. Your thoughts about the brownie are the problem.

Demand of yourself the self-awareness that comes from honesty. Stop thinking in incomplete thoughts. Saying *I already blew it, so what's the point?* is an incomplete thought you choose, a lie you tell yourself because it's easy, convenient, and familiar. Commit to the entire story.

What is the point?

Did you blow it?

What does blowing it mean?

Is there a problem?

What's the solution?

Can you make it better?

How?

Can you make it worse?

How?

If you convince yourself to make more of the same choices, what happens?

How will that make you feel?

Is it worth it?

Think about how catastrophic and inconceivable all-or-nothing thinking would be in any other area of your life.

I'm late to pick up the kids, so what's the point? I'll leave them there and try to be on time tomorrow.

I'm late on this project deadline, so screw it. I'll take the day off and try again tomorrow.

The consequences would be disastrous.

They're presently disastrous.

As you become increasingly aware of the ways you negotiate for the permission to be "off" or choose "nothing," you can begin to practice an alternative approach.

An alternative to all-or-nothing lives in the middle. **Pursue the middle.**

Instead of thinking that you either make it to the gym today or you do nothing, what is the middle ground? What are all the options that live between the workout you intended and doing nothing?

Instead of thinking that you either eat perfectly or you

binge, what's in the middle? What are all the options that live between the two ends of the spectrum?

Identify the middle options and choose them. Do you see that these changes in behavior stem from changes in your thoughts? Commit to practice.

QUESTIONS TO ASK

- What behaviors both predict and influence the goal you want to achieve?
- How can you focus today on changing your thoughts about your challenges or goals?
- Where are you telling incomplete truths to justify all-or-nothing behaviors?
- What is the whole truth you're avoiding?
- What happens when you choose an all-or-nothing approach?
- What do you know about what doesn't work for you?
- How can you avoid approaches that don't work?
- What's a middle ground between your excuse and your intention?

EIGHT

External Goals and Internal Targets

"The grass isn't greener in the other field...the experience you experience is traveling with you."

—GURU SINGH

I used to watch NBC's hit television show *The Biggest Loser* and *wish* for the "opportunity" to live on the Biggest Loser Ranch, where my entire life could revolve around weight loss.

It seemed like a dream scenario that would make all my problems disappear.

I'd tell myself, "If I didn't have to worry about work, avoiding temptations, or making time to work out, I'd totally conquer my weight issue!"

I would have given just about anything to live in that bubble, certain that if my sole focus were weight loss, I would make it happen. Beyond that, I was convinced that losing weight would make me happy. I really believed that I wasn't happy because I was overweight, and therefore, if I wasn't overweight, I'd be happy.

Maybe you've had similar thoughts. If you worked in a gym and could work out all day like that super-fit trainer you know, you'd be fit, too. If you made that six-figure salary, you wouldn't be stressed about money.

Here's what those thoughts overlook: **your primary barriers to change aren't external, they're internal.**

The primary issue isn't outside you, it's *inside* you.

Your primary barriers aren't your job, finances, or lack of free time. You can convince yourself that these external circumstances remove or reduce your power to choose, but that's not actually true. Believing in a barrier doesn't make it real. You can make a great choice when you're short on time, patience, or money. The opportunity is never removed because of your physical or emotional resources.

Most of us are quick to tell ourselves that our external conditions dictate our internal conditions. We're stressed because of our jobs. We're tired because of our schedule. We're overweight because of life stress or constant travel and temptations.

In truth, it's the other way around. **Our internal conditions create our external conditions.**

Said another way, we're not unhappy because we're overweight; we're overweight because we're unhappy. We aren't depressed because we drink too much; we drink too much because we're depressed.

Why do the vast majority of contestants on *The Biggest Loser* regain the weight? Why do people who win the lottery end up wasting away their windfall?

Because, like the rest of us, their primary barriers are *also* internal. When they return to their normal settings, they struggle with the same internal barriers they had before.

Changing the external conditions might allow for temporary progress, but *permanent* progress requires that you get to the root of the issue: the internal barriers.

Real life isn't lived in a bubble like the one often created for television. In the isolation of the Biggest Loser Ranch, contestants optimize their external conditions, but rarely their internal ones. They aren't forced to do the critical work of overcoming excuses and exceptions and managing emotional triggers. All of those real-life hurdles are cleared for them.

If that show taught me anything, it's that there are no shortcuts. The Biggest Loser Ranch is not a shortcut. At best, it's a detour. As is always the case, the *real work* must be done for the results to be sustained.

The same is true when people win the lottery. Sure, it sounds nice, right? It's easy to think it would solve so many of your problems. But most people who win the lottery blow through the money and not only fail to maintain the wealth they won, but end up with *more* financial hardship *after* the lottery than they had before.

Why? Because the experience you experience travels with you. More money, same problems. Or, less weight, same problems.

In order to identify the work you truly need to focus on and ensure that you are making lasting progress toward your goal, it's critical that you get crystal clear on *why* you want to achieve the goal. The *why* is often overlooked and taken for granted but it's actually the most important aspect of pursuing change. It's perceived as less important touchy-feely stuff.

It's essential. I wish someone had explained this to me decades ago—it has made a massive difference in my life.

I need you to trust me when I tell you that it's not enough to know *what* you want. Being able to articulate what you want is entirely incomplete. We can't be sure of your personal path to change until we've fully explored *why* you want to create the change.

Even if you *think* you know why you want this goal, I can assure you that there's work to be done in articulating the why behind the what. Almost without fail, my clients struggle to define their *why*.

Just to make sure you're tracking with me, let me put it a different way. When I talk about the *why* behind the goal, I'm asking you to consider what will be different about your life when you have achieved it. We're differentiating between external goals and internal targets. What will be different about how you feel or how you don't feel? The external change is obvious, but what is the internal change you're seeking?

What is it that you'll be, have, experience, or feel when you've achieved your goal that you don't have now?

I had to learn this the hard way. One of the primary reasons I struggled with my weight for so long was that I didn't know *why* I was trying to lose weight or *what*, other than less fatness, I was pursuing. In fact, I will argue strongly that if someone helped me get clear on *why* I wanted to lose weight much earlier in life, I would have avoided decades of yo-yo dieting and weight gain.

My external goal was crystal clear: I wanted to lose weight.

I couldn't help but wonder why, if I truly wanted to lose weight so badly, I'd keep quitting diets and returning right back to overeating after successfully losing a few pounds. If I wanted to lose weight so badly, why did I keep choosing food, knowing full well I couldn't eat that way *and* lose weight?

It's not that I loved food more than I desired weight loss; most of the food I was eating wasn't even that great.

I certainly wasn't alone. If people are so desperate for weight loss, why are they so quick to put weight back on? Why do people return to alcohol after fighting so hard for sobriety?

Believe it or not, it's not because people are weak. In fact, most of us are far stronger than we give ourselves credit for.

The powerful truth lies in the fact that most people aren't clear on the thing they want most.

I didn't know what my internal targets were. And to be honest, I didn't think they mattered. I just wanted to lose weight because I was fat. That's all. The problem was fatness; the solution was less fatness. I hadn't really thought about what would be different or better about my life when I lost the weight, but hidden in those considerations was the key to creating sustainable change.

In 2014, I was attending a conference for female business owners. During a lecture on self-acceptance, I sat in the back of the room, last seat, last row. In most settings, I prefer to be a wallflower and not draw attention to myself. During this talk, the speaker was trying to make the case that we are perfect as we are and do not need to change.

I'm sorry, what? It didn't jive with me. The idea alone made me defensive and uncomfortable. At that point in my own journey, I had lost about one hundred pounds but still considered myself overweight, and was eager to continue my physical transformation.

The idea of accepting myself felt like settling for less than my potential. It felt like surrender. It felt like quitting or letting myself off the hook. I didn't understand why we'd be encouraged to accept ourselves as is and resist the desire to change. Wasn't that the opposite of drive and ambition? Shouldn't we *want* to get better?

I'm totally on board for not hating yourself, but simple acceptance? Surrendering drive? He lost me.

I'm not one to raise my hand or speak up in a group, but I couldn't resist.

I don't remember exactly what I said, but it went a little something like this:

"Isn't it good to want to change? Isn't it part of how we drive growth and improvement in our lives? How is acceptance different from settling?"

I'll give the man credit. It's never easy to have someone question your approach in front of a roomful of people. He did a great job of directing his inquiry to me specifically, instead of speaking in generalities, but he still didn't convince me.

He asked me what I wanted to change about myself and I answered honestly, even though I felt embarrassed to say it out loud, as though the room wasn't able to see my size until I said the words out loud. I wanted to lose more weight.

He asked me why I felt my weight was a problem. Why did I feel I needed to change? I was confused. He could *see* that I was overweight. Wasn't that enough? What other reason could there be?

I wish it had been a red flag for me then that I couldn't articulate why I wanted to lose weight, but it wasn't. All I knew was that I simply didn't want to be overweight anymore. He kept returning to the questions, "What is the problem? Why do you have to change?" I had no answer other than "I'm fat."

Eventually, my embarrassment and frustration reached an unfortunate crescendo and I stood up, grabbed my thighs, and said, "*These* are the problem! This is why I want to change!"

Awkward giggles filled the room. Though, to a small extent, I was using humor and dramatics to ease the tension I was feeling, it wasn't a funny moment.

I wish I could tell you that he helped me create a breakthrough that day, but he didn't. I can see, in hindsight, that he was *trying* to take me there, but either he didn't show me the right path or I wasn't willing to take it. Probably a little of both.

I wish he had asked me, "Elizabeth, what is it that you want that you don't have? What will you have when you lose weight that you don't have now? What will you have more of? What will you have less of?"

Those were questions I hadn't considered but would find transformative in the years to come.

Clearly, there was more to my goal than simply wanting to weigh less because, even after losing weight, becoming debt-free, and launching a business, I was *still* unhappy. I was still depressed and my marriage got worse, not better.

Here's what I probably would have said, had he asked those questions.

"I want to feel great about my body. I want to feel confident. I don't want to feel like I'm fighting against myself. I want to feel at peace, not emotionally burdened by my body. I want to genuinely *want* to eat well. I don't want to feel drawn to things that make me feel awful, like binging."

There they are...my internal targets.

I had lost one hundred pounds but I didn't feel any more confident. Why did I think that twenty or thirty pounds more would make a difference? We all know many lean people who lack confidence. **It wasn't my body that created my lack of confidence; it was my thoughts about my body.**

It wasn't my size that made me feel like I was fighting against myself; it was my perspective.

Being overweight didn't create emotional turmoil. My thoughts about being overweight did.

It started to become clear to me that it wasn't so much about wanting to be a certain size; I wanted to feel a certain way that I thought would automatically result from being a certain size.

I wanted to be at peace with my body and feel confident. I felt that more weight loss would create that, but it's not true. Confidence and peace of mind are not gifts bestowed upon the lean. External goals do not hit internal targets.

I had some internal work to do. The clarity that came with identifying my internal targets and the why behind my desire to lose weight made my journey much easier.

I started to realize that the reason I hadn't magically become confident after losing weight had nothing to do with the weight loss and everything to do with my thoughts.

I began asking myself, "What will make me feel more confident? What can I do about it today? What makes me feel less confident? What can I do about it today?"

Sometimes, the steps I took to create confidence had nothing to do with the steps I took to lose weight. Often, they overlapped. Either way, I was pursuing both aims this time, not just one.

Hitting external goals will not change your internal conditions.

Changing your body will not change your mindset about your body.

Changing your bank balance will not change your thoughts about money.

External goals cannot hit internal targets.

"The grass isn't greener in the other field...the experience you are experiencing travels with you."

This quote from Guru Singh describes the point we're chasing here. If you're unhappy when you're heavy, you'll still be unhappy when you're not as heavy.

If you're anxious when you're broke, you'll be anxious when you have money.

If you're depressed in this job, you'll be depressed in the next.

The experience travels with you. Your perspective and mindset travel with you.

You must identify your internal target so you can proceed more effectively and avoid continuing to be unfulfilled even after achieving that thing you think you want. It's a deeply empty way to live, chasing the wrong goal and remaining dissatisfied.

SMOKE OR FIRE?

Let's talk about you and *your* goals.

Right now, you're likely pursuing an external goal because you think it will help you hit an internal target.

This often looks like pursuing weight loss because you think it will make you happier or more confident, or pursuing debt reduction because you think it will make you less stressed.

Weight loss and less debt are external goals.

Happiness, confidence, and peace of mind are internal targets.

The external targets are *absolutely* worthy of being pursued; I just want to help you make sure you're also pursuing that internal target separately, so you don't find yourself unfulfilled after putting in all that time and effort.

It's important to note that your external goal is often associated with an internal issue. For example, obesity is rarely just about eating too much. Eating too much is often a symptom stemming from an internal issue like insecurity, depression, or sadness. Food is often an escape or a distraction. It's often an anesthetic, a way for you to avoid feeling something else. What lies beneath?

The same is true with people who struggle to manage their finances. Overspending is rarely about the material things people collect. Spending is often a symptom of an internal problem like anxiety or loneliness. Spending can be a way of creating a moment of pleasure and confusing it with happiness.

To understand the power of this shift in your thinking, I'd like you to think of your challenges and struggles as either smoke or fire.

As you know, smoke and fire are two very different things, and confusing them can be disastrous.

If you're trying to fight a fire, you cannot succeed by merely addressing the smoke. It's impossible. You must find the fire and extinguish it. Yes, the smoke can cause problems, but the smoke isn't *the* problem. You can't eliminate the smoke until you extinguish the fire.

Another way to distinguish between your external goals and internal targets is to differentiate between the smoke and the fires in your life.

If you busy yourself trying to clear the smoke, your work will never be done. The smoke remains until the fire is extinguished. For me, my weight was the smoke. Low self-esteem was the fire. I had to address the fire to effectively create change.

When it comes to your goals, the smoke could be overeating, excessive drinking, spending, gossiping, or complaining. The smoke is coming from the fire.

More often than not, our external goals address the smoke, but not the fire.

Where's the fire?

The fire is usually an internal issue: low self-esteem, loneliness, unhappiness, stress, anxiety, or fear.

When we do the work to identify why we want to achieve these external goals, we're heading toward the fire.

External goals can't hit internal targets, just like clearing the smoke won't put out a fire.

As we move through this chapter I'll be giving you tools, considerations, and questions to help you distinguish between your external goal and internal targets.

Health or happiness?

When I'm working with clients, I talk a lot about choosing happiness as the path to health instead of health as the path to happiness.

I know I wasn't alone when I thought that if I could just lose the weight, everything would be better. I definitely believed that weight loss would make me happier.

I believed paying off debt would make me happier.

Many people believe that drinking less or saving more money will make them happier.

The problem is, it's not the weight or the debt or the drinking that makes you unhappy. It's a combination of your thoughts about those things and the factors driving the weight, the debt, or the drinking.

I'm here to help you break that line of thinking and flip

it on its head and pursue happiness (or another internal target) as the primary goal and the external goals as separate endeavors.

The fact of the matter is that happier people take better care of themselves. They aren't looking for an escape or soothing via food, alcohol, or spending.

Put the internal target ahead of the external goal. You'll save a lot of time and energy that way. You'll find that your achievement isn't so hollow and you won't continue to wrestle with the same external problems for years or decades.

It's completely okay if you can't initially pinpoint your internal targets. For years, you've focused on the external goal.

I used to have a really hard time identifying how I wanted to feel. For quite a while, I could only tell you how I *didn't* want to feel. That's a fantastic start. Begin there.

Growing up, people used to say to me, "Nothing tastes as good as thin feels!"

Well, I had never been thin; I didn't understand. I couldn't get excited about that. I still cringe every time I see those words.

I didn't know what it felt like to walk into a store and be able to try on anything. I didn't know what it felt like to fly on an airplane without worrying that the seatbelt wouldn't fit. I didn't know what it felt like to look in the mirror naked and love what I saw or be with a person who thought I was sexy and didn't want me to change. It's really hard to be motivated by something you've never come close to experiencing, so you're not alone if you feel that way.

I had to take a smaller step and a simpler approach.

I simply started to evaluate what choices made me unhappy.

I asked myself questions like:

- When do I feel bad?
- What choices make me feel bad?
- How can I minimize those things today?
- What do I want to feel less of?
- What can I do about it today?

The first rule of holes is "stop digging."

If you can identify what choices **don't** give you what you want and what choices make you unhappy, that's a powerful place to start.

Ask yourself how you will avoid those things today.

Keep that first rule of holes top of mind. Keep that list of things that make life worse, increase your stress, or make you unhappy top of mind. Write it in your phone or trigger it to be sent to you as an email every day.

For those of you who struggle to find these answers, I want to share with you some of mine. I'm certain that my answers won't be your answers, but I know how it feels to just not know. Use these as a starting point for creating your own progress.

What choices erode my happiness, confidence, or peace of mind?

- Breaking promises I make to myself or others
- Overeating
- Sleeping too much
- Not sleeping enough
- Not taking care of the space around me
- Complaining
- Focusing on my problems (versus focusing on my solutions)
- Blaming other people
- Isolating myself and avoiding social situations
- Beating myself up over the past
- Giving my energy to fear of the future

What choices increase my happiness, inner peace, confidence, or clarity?

- Working out
- Keeping my home clean
- Being intentional about building relationships with people close to me
- Budgeting and keeping good financial records
- Meditation
- Gratitude
- Journaling
- Eating well
- Going to bed early
- Getting up early
- Saying "no thank you" to alcohol and indulgences

What about you?

QUESTIONS TO ASK

- What is it that you'll have, be, experience, or feel when you reach your goal that you don't have now?
- What do you want to feel that you don't feel now?
- What do you want more of in your life?
- What do you want less of?
- What contributes to happiness?
- What contributes to unhappiness?
- What makes you feel calm?

- What arouses stress or anxiety?
- What are your internal goals?
- What are your external targets?
- What can you do to pursue that internal target separately instead of assuming it will come along with the achievement of the external goal?
- When you get to the end of your life, how would you have to live to consider it a great success?
- How do you define a happy life?
- What are the gaps between that happy life you've defined and the life you're living now?
- What can you do today to begin to bridge the gap?

NINE

Customer Service Is an Inside Job

After a few seconds of focusing on the problem, you are best served to move to the solution. Don't stay with the problem beyond the point of establishing an understanding of it.

I don't read a lot of magazines. In fact, I only have one current magazine subscription and it's to the *Harvard Business Review*.

I find an inspiring number of parallels between the strategies that create success in business and the tactics that create success in life.

There was an article in the January/February 2018 issue called "'Sorry' Is Not Enough"* that helped me understand the requirements for creating change more clearly.

---

* "Sorry Is Not Enough," *Harvard Business Review*, January/February 2018, https://hbr.org/2018/01/sorry-is-not-enough.

The article was looking at the types of customer service approaches that drive the most satisfaction (and dissatisfaction) when customers are facing a service problem. The researchers reviewed a series of service experiences within the airline industry.

I was immediately intrigued, not because I have a passion for the customer service industry, but because at its most basic level, like creating personal change, customer service is about overcoming challenges and solving problems.

I'm sure you've had a less-than-stellar experience with an airline—maybe your flight was cancelled or your bags were lost. In those moments, what do you want? Would you rather have an apology from an empathetic airline representative or have a creative, energetic problem solver take concrete **action steps that resolve your problem?** I think most of us want the latter. Sure, empathy feels nice but it doesn't get us anywhere. You want the problem solved as quickly and pleasantly as possible.

The researchers categorized the responses from airline representatives as either **relational work** or **problem-solving work.**

Relational work includes things like listening to the customer's complaints, apologizing, empathizing, and expressing understanding. "I understand you're frustrated. I'm sorry. We'll get you out of here as soon as we can. My sister's flight was cancelled last month and it delayed her vacation; I know how upsetting this can be."

Problem-solving work is any attempt to deliver a solution. "Here are our options: we can get you on a flight to a different hub and still have you make your connection, or I can get you on the first flight tomorrow and provide you with a $500 credit and hotel accommodations for this evening."

I wasn't surprised by one of the article's conclusions:

"An apology that extends beyond the first seconds of an interaction can reduce customer satisfaction. Employees should instead focus on **demonstrating how creatively and energetically they are trying to solve the customer's problem.**"

I doubt you're surprised either.

But let's *not* just nod in obvious agreement and rush along. There's so much we can take from that simple statement when we break it down. What we take from it can dramatically improve *your* ability to create change and help you identify ways you are holding yourself back so you can more effectively participate in creating solutions.

It doesn't help much if the airline agent dives deeper into the problem after the core of the issue has been identified. "Trying to get to Omaha, huh? I've never been there. What's in Omaha? Business or pleasure?"

Who cares? Get me there!

That might seem obvious in customer service, but **we often ignore the obvious necessity of moving quickly from the problem to the solution in our own lives.**

We spend far too long thinking about, complaining about, and rehashing the problem long after we have enough information to proceed to the solution. We take an unnecessarily long and deep dive into the problem and our feelings about it than is helpful.

As the article suggests, after *a few seconds* of empathy, once a baseline understanding has been established, you are best served to move to a solution.

There's more. The researchers don't *just* suggest quickly moving from relational work to problem-solving work.

"Employees should instead **demonstrate** how...they are trying to solve the problem."

The word "demonstrate" is critical. **Demonstration**

requires action. Satisfactory outcomes require that we not only identify solutions, but *act on them*.

You must **move quickly** from the problem **to taking action** on the solution.

It's **not** that you move quickly to *talking or thinking* about the solution. You need to move quickly to *demonstrating* your participation in the solution. Do something. Participate. Be the change. Remember the "hard road" we keep talking about? That's the one where you spin in circles around the problem and thinking about the solution without taking consistent action.

The easier road is the direct path straight from identifying the problem to taking action on the solution.

After all, transformation is **now**.

There's another game-changing part of the article's conclusion that makes a world of difference, and it's the words **"creatively"** and **"energetically."**

"Employees should instead focus on **demonstrating** how **creatively** and **energetically** they are trying to solve the customer's problem."

Wouldn't you love to have customer service representatives creatively and energetically take action to solve your problems? I know I would!

That is precisely how you should tackle your *own* problems: creatively and energetically. After all, this is your life! Quite frankly, the problem keeping you from your best life or healthiest self is certainly more deserving of creative, energetic problem-solving than your cancelled flight, erroneous cable bill, or broken washing machine, right?

What if you employed this approach in your own life? How different would your experience of challenges, setbacks, or past patterns be if instead of spending hours, weeks, or even years being a victim of your problems or crushed by your circumstances you simply committed to creatively and energetically taking action on solutions?

What if you took that approach with your health, your work, your finances, and your relationships? What a different experience of "problems" you would have! Moreover, you'd probably be infinitely happier and less stressed.

For nearly the first thirty years of my life, I **only** did that relational work. I wasn't doing much problem-solving work, I wasn't taking much action, and I certainly wasn't a creative, energetic problem solver on my own behalf. Not even close. I complained about my weight.

I complained about eating healthy. I complained about eating unhealthy. I complained about my job, my lack of friends, and my unhappiness. I created a sense of powerlessness—I felt like my past patterns, habits, and circumstances had more power over my ability to change than I did. I convinced myself that I was the victim.

Nothing could be further from the truth, for me and for you, but if you're choosing to limit yourself to relational work, you'll convince yourself of that, too.

Don't get me wrong: I still have problems. Lots of them. Every day. And I still have days where those problems feel bigger and stronger than the solutions. While the problems are real, my ability to choose to demonstrate creative, energetic problem-solving is just as real, and certainly far more productive and effective.

This life is short, my potential is real, and I deserve to provide myself with that degree of energy and creativity.

You do, too.

SENSING OR SOLVING?

Though I'd have been grateful if *that* mindset shift was all I got from the HBR customer service article, there was much more.

The researchers divided interactions with customers into three phases: sensing, seeking, and settling.

In the sensing phase, representatives ask questions to understand the totality of the issue.

In the seeking phase, they brainstorm and explore potential solutions.

Finally, in the settling phase, they choose a resolution that will provide the best outcome.

I recently had a customer service experience, and I took the opportunity to recognize each of these phases.

As I was finishing up the manuscript for this book, I decided to rent an oceanfront house for a week. I wanted a pleasant change of scenery for long days of writing.

One morning, I started to prepare a recipe I wanted to post on my blog, only to find that the gas stove wouldn't light. After messing with it, I decided to wait for my boyfriend to return and take a look.

A couple hours later, I jumped into the shower only to realize there was no hot water.

Fantastic. The gas had been turned off! I called the

rental agency and informed them of the problem. They called back with some bad news: the gas bill hadn't been paid in months, so the gas company had come out and shut it off. Moreover, they couldn't turn it back on for two days.

The sensing phase of our customer service interaction involved us getting on the same page about the problem: no hot water, no stove, no dryer.

In the seeking phase, she explained our options. They would restore gas service two days later and credit me for the days without gas or, instead of money, we could extend our stay by a few days.

In the settling phase, I accepted the offer to extend our stay.

Based on best practice and an awareness of what creates the greatest degree of customer satisfaction, the article ends with the following recommendation:

"Just get into the task and generate interesting options for the customer."

Get into the task and generate interesting options. Get to work and be creative in the solutions you consider and pursue.

What if you did that in your own life? What if, after identifying the problem, you creatively and energetically generated options for yourself? What if you quickly got to work demonstrating your commitment to the solution? What if you made that your simple, nonnegotiable operating system? It would be a game changer.

You'd make more progress, spend less time feeling sorry for yourself, and avoid needless (unproductive) worry about the problems and the past.

You will save infinite amounts of time, energy, and emotion when you implement this strategy.

While this sensing, seeking, settling framework is undoubtedly a great start, it is missing one critical piece:

ACTION.

I'm a sucker for things that are easy to remember so I'll stick with the HBR article's "s" words naming convention. We'll call that missing piece "solving."

Here's how I want to amend and help you adopt this framework so you can practice implementing it in your life:

Sensing

Seeking

Settling

Solving

Let's take a closer look at how you can leverage this structure for faster results with less effort, less time, and less emotion. You might see that skipping one of these steps, or spending too much time in one of them, is one of the things holding you back from creating the change you crave.

This will be how we take another turn off that hard road and avoid the white-knuckle approach.

SENSING

There is an undeniable necessity for the sensing phase— asking questions to understand the situation, problem, or challenge. What happened? What's wrong? What's the behavior you want to change? What is the problem you're looking to solve? In the sensing phase, you get a **base level** understanding for the challenge and the circumstances surrounding it.

Remember: don't let this phase extend too long. **Move**

quickly to the solution. Once you're clear on what the problem is, it's time to move to the next phase.

You don't need to linger and obsess over seven thousand layers of understanding and analysis.

One hole a lot of people dig for themselves is a result of **not moving out of the sensing stage.** They want to get a PhD in the psychology of the problem. Not necessary. You don't need five years of therapy, thirty-eight books, eighteen hours of audio, a thirty-day plan and sixteen thousand conversations to get clear on an action step you can take to demonstrate creative, energetic problem-solving.

Just like the airline attendant doesn't need to ask twenty questions about why you're headed to Omaha and if the trip is for business or pleasure, you too need to skip the tendency to spin your wheels in the analysis of the problem and its many considerations.

Don't give all your energy to the problem. Don't even give it the majority of your energy. You don't have to stay in your feelings about an issue. Don't be owned by your feelings. Give your energy to the solution.

Identify the problem, establish a base level of understanding, and *move quickly* to the next stage.

SEEKING

Seeking is the natural next step. Brainstorm and explore all your potential options for creating a solution or making progress toward a different result.

Remember the questions I asked my client about her emotional eating? What else is true? What are the other options you have? I used this strategy in coming up with a different way to respond to the noisy Starbucks and sitting in traffic.

Don't skip this step. *Resist the temptation to move automatically to the solution you've always tried*, especially if that one isn't working! Yes, there's a most-familiar response, but it's not the only option. Acknowledge them all.

Keep that Charlie Munger quote in mind: "To a man with a hammer, everything looks like a nail." The answer isn't always work harder, restrict more, or try again with that thing that never works.

There will be an undeniable pull toward the familiar, but resist that perceived shortcut. It's no shortcut at all. You are here to explore all the options, not just the first ones that come to your mind.

I recently heard someone say that **"binary" is the opposite of "creativity."**

Binary means having two parts. Think of it as "it's this way or it's that way." It's left or right. Black or white. All-or-nothing. Binge or restrict. Yes or no.

Those perspectives are the *opposite* of creativity, because there are almost always many, many options you've overlooked and you're simply limiting yourself to the most extreme or the most familiar.

I see this all the time when people are trying to get healthy or lose weight. They're either on a diet or they're off. They're either being super disciplined in how they eat or they're going hog wild and enjoying whatever they want, whenever they want, as much as they want.

Sure, those are two options, but they aren't the *only* two options. Not even close. When you opt for a binary perspective, you opt *out* of creative problem-solving.

When you're in the seeking phase, make sure you avoid binary thinking.

What are all the possible options? What are all the different ways you could solve this or create progress and change?

SETTLING

It's decision time. In the settling phase, you decide on a course of action.

Of all the possible solutions you considered, which is the one you're able and willing to act on...today?

That last word is the most important one: today. **Settling isn't a religion.** You aren't bound to this decision until the end of time.

Your bandwidth and ability to initiate change varies from day to day. Plus, you're learning as you go, so allow for change without rigidity. Don't take on the future; only take on the present. You don't have to figure out your strategy for eternity, or even for the next week.

Identifying actions you're able to take today makes change less overwhelming and more immediate.

Be honest about today's solution and demand of yourself that you follow through, just for today.

WHEN YOU FEEL STUCK

The next stage is the one I added to the HBR article, and I think it's the most important one. Before we talk about

solving, I want to bring your attention to why change feels so hard as it relates to the first three stages.

Most people get stuck in a cycle of sensing the problem, seeking solutions, settling on one, and then going right back into sensing or seeking without shifting energy and consistency to solving.

You've probably experienced it more than once. It looks something like this:

You're aware of the problem. You think about it all the time. You beat yourself up. You're mad about it. You wish things were different. You know what you're doing is wrong, you know when you do it, and you know many (if not all) of the factors that drive you to it. A lot of time goes into that sensing stage.

Then, you focus on solutions. You read all the books and the blogs. You talk about it with your friends. You ask what they're doing. You keep an eye on their results, or lack thereof. You ask Google for plans and strategies. What are the best practices? You listen to podcasts and maybe even buy courses or products. Time, energy, effort, and emotion pour into seeking.

You've probably settled, too. You make up your mind: I'm going to make a change. Monday is the day. I'm serious this time. No excuses. I'm tired of this struggle. You commit to a plan, program, or approach. All those declarations and well-intended commitments fall into the settling stage.

However, the solving doesn't follow the decision. If it does, it doesn't last long, you stop short of consistency, and then go right back to sensing or seeking. You go right back into your feelings or considering other options, shortcutting what is required for change: consistent action.

Many people cycle through sensing, seeking, and settling without moving (and staying) in the solving stage. They move from their feelings about the problem to planning to take action, deciding what action to take, failing to act, and right back into their feelings.

Solving is action. Solving requires participation in the creation of the solution.

All the other stages are either related to the problem and how you feel about it or theorizing about possible solutions.

To create lasting change, the majority of your time and energy needs to be spent, creatively and energetically, in the solving stage.

If you're struggling to create change, take a look at where

most of your time, energy, effort, and emotion are going. Chances are, it's not in solving—it's not in action.

Do not be subject to inertia. Inertia is a tendency to do nothing or remain unchanged. Recognize when you're in this phase of not taking action. Thinking isn't acting. **Giving time to the problem isn't the same as giving energy to the solution.**

For most of my life, I thought I was solving my problems because I *wanted* to solve them and I spent so much time and energy seeking solutions. I was spinning my wheels, getting nowhere, giving myself credit for my intentions.

I was beyond frustrated by my weight. I was exhausted by the struggle. I hated my body. I felt mentally weak and physically exhausted. I was ashamed. Often, I was straight-up furious with myself for failing to execute. I was resentful of my past and fearful of my future. I was hiding from my friends and family because I was embarrassed by my size and failure to change. Most of my thoughts and emotions were locked up in **sensing**.

I was the ultimate seeker. I walked away from my Latin scholarship and dream of being a lawyer to study nutrition because I was desperate for answers. I worked in the nutrition industry. I read every diet book and followed dozens of health blogs. I spent an embarrassing amount of time **seeking** information and potential solutions.

Every week I was **settling** on a new solution. *Atkins! I'm all in. I'm serious this time. Wait, no. I'm going to count calories. The stricter the better! No more sugar for me! I've had enough sugar to last me the rest of my life and I am committing to whole foods only! For life! You know, on second thought, I should just hire a personal trainer. If I'm working out regularly, I'm sure that will motivate me to eat better.*

None of those strategies mattered a bit without a commitment to solving and determined, regular action on the steps of the solution. **Nothing** changed in my life until I decided to be a problem solver. Nothing changed until **I decided to take unyielding action on the result I wanted to produce.** I had to borrow some energy from all the thinking and feeling so I had some to give to action.

I'm going to give you 100,000 bonus points if you've wondered, "Wait. Elizabeth, you said thinking was the most important place to start creating change. But now you're saying action is the only thing that drives change. Which is it? Do I want to get out of the sensing phase and into the solving phase or do I really want to focus on my thoughts?"

I'm so glad you asked!

As soon as you are clear on the problem, get to the action. The important part about changing how you think is that you have the ability to train yourself to think about the solution instead of the problem.

Changing your thoughts allows you to shift from "I can't" to "How can I?" You're shifting your thoughts in a way that allows you to more effectively (and quickly) participate in the solution.

Optimizing the way you think allows you to take the right action to create change instead of taking no change or creating more of the problem.

Action is the antidote.

SOLVING

Solving is action. It's demonstration. It's the only thing that drives results. It's not a *decision* to act; it's getting off the sidelines, getting into the game, and *doing* something.

The efficacy of everything else depends on the time, effort, and consistency you invest in solving.

Solving is making that improved choice. Saying "no" when you want to say "yes" and saying "yes" when you want to say "no." Solving is *being* the change.

Solving is living "transformation is now" as your operating system. Solving means choosing transformation, moment after moment, understanding and leveraging the reality that every choice is a chance to create the change you crave.

Shifting into the mode of solving and out of the other categories requires that you understand what it looks like, for you, to *be* in each of these categories.

Here are some examples of thoughts, patterns, and behaviors in each area.

Sensing: guilt; regret; fear; anxiety; comparison; hope; anticipation; past patterns; past experiences; future events; making excuses; negotiating exceptions.

You know you're sensing when your thoughts and words are about how you feel about yourself, your problem, your fears, your past, or your future. Sensing includes positive, negative, and neutral thoughts and feelings.

Seeking: reading books; listening to podcasts; researching; searching online for ideas, answers, or understanding; following blogs or social media personalities; asking for expert (and nonexpert) opinions.

You know you are seeking when your thoughts, words, or

actions are about obtaining more information or considering possible solutions.

Settling: committing to a new approach, program, plan, behavior, pattern, or habit. Planning and strategizing are settling activities.

You know you are settling when you are pledging to a new plan, behavior, or habit but you're focused on the decision versus acting on the decision. You know you're settling when you're clear on the problem and the potential solution but you aren't doing anything about it, or you aren't taking action consistently. Settling includes committing to a solution but failing to implement it.

Solving: taking an action that delivers the change you want to create. **It's not a plan to act; it's a choice or behavior that produces a direct result.** This could be making a healthy meal, turning down dessert, completing a workout, cutting unnecessary expenses, or meditating. Solving will look very different depending on your individual goal.

Solving is action-oriented. You aren't thinking about the solution, you are actively creating it. You're taking action on what you can do right now to create the outcome you want.

Creating change isn't a sprint. The winner isn't the one who goes the fastest; it's the one who doesn't stop.

IS IT A DREAM OR A GOAL?

It might be helpful to consider if the change you want to create is a dream or a goal. Dreams are aspirational, but that doesn't mean we're taking action to bring them into reality. When you have a goal, you plan on achieving it. You're going to do what it takes to make it happen. Don't confuse dreams and goals.

There are plenty of people who dream of being wealthy but don't have intentions of putting forth consistent effort to make it happen.

You can turn any dream into a goal. Don't give up or give in because answers or strategies don't come easily to you. Backing off might feel more comfortable in the moment, but it only compounds the problem.

This is where you need to lean in, not pull away. Remember that what you put in to changing the way you think and creating change in your life determines what you'll get out of it.

Transformation is now. Embrace this moment when you feel frustrated or uncertain and be the change right now.

You don't have to wait. What you do today matters. It makes a difference. Everything you do makes a difference.

RECOVER QUICKLY

There's a term in the fitness world called the refractory period. The refractory period refers to the span of time after a muscle is stimulated when it recovers before further stimulation. If your eyebrow is raised because you think of refractory period in terms of sex, you're not wrong! The refractory period is also the time frame between orgasm and when you feel capable of getting busy again.

This concept is actually a great one to help you get back into action in your own life.

I want you to think about the span of time between a choice you *aren't* proud of and a choice you *are* proud of as your refractory period.

How can you shorten the refractory period?

Let's say you are on your third glass of wine. In the past, maybe you've used that to justify pizza, dessert, and a cocktail. You figure you've blown the night, so what's the point?

The span of time between that third glass of wine and

your next great choice is your refractory period. How can you make it shorter?

How quickly can you get to your next great choice?

Instead of taking a day or two to bounce back, challenge yourself to get to your next great choice as quickly as possible.

But change is a result of practicing the change, not deciding on it.

The next time you make a choice that you don't feel proud of, see how quickly you can get back to great choices that make you feel your best. Did you overdo it on the pizza? Close the kitchen for the night, have a glass of water, and head to bed. Did you go bananas at the dessert table during the office luncheon? Head right to the gym from work. Maybe you snapped at your spouse—pick up the phone and apologize instead of being passive-aggressive all night long. Choose to make that refractory period as short as possible!

IT'S YOUR TURN

Take a minute to identify how sensing, seeking, settling, and solving show up in your life. Take a minute to fill out the chart below as it relates to an area of your life where you're struggling to create change.

Complete the chart with the thoughts, behaviors, words, and patterns that reflect each of these previously described stages.

For example, if the change you want to create is weight loss, sensing might include beating yourself up for last night's choices or worrying about the ten pounds you want to lose before the holidays. Seeking might be the time you spend reading or listening to podcasts. Settling might be your Sunday night commitment to eating clean this week, and solving is choosing to eat steak and salad after rejecting Chinese takeout.

If the change you want to create is related to paying down debt, your sensing activities might include stressing over how you're going to pay your bills. Seeking might include reading up on strategies for paying down debt or looking for a cheaper apartment. Settling could include your frequent pledges to cut back on your spending. Solving could include getting a second job or calling to cancel your cable.

Now it's your turn.

Once you've gone through each area, honestly evaluate where you're prone to spend the most time and energy.

CATEGORY	THOUGHTS, PATTERNS, BEHAVIORS
SENSING	
SEEKING	
SETTLING	
SOLVING	

When you feel stuck or overwhelmed, I want you to return to *your* chart to assess where you can be a better steward of your time and attention.

You can be a creative, energetic problem solver, and it begins by identifying what action you can take now and next to move in the direction of your goals.

You are now clearer on the right work you need to do to create the change you crave. But knowing the right work doesn't equip you to actually do it.

QUESTIONS TO ASK

- To what problems are you not applying creative, energetic solutions?
- On what problems can you practice?
- If someone else were in charge of solving the problems in your life—if it was their actions and energy that made the difference—how would you want them to show up? What would you want them to do?
- How can you be *more* creative and energetic in the way you solve problems in your life?
- In which of the phases of the problem do you feel you are wasting energy: sensing, seeking, settling, or solving?
- Where do you need to spend more time?
- How can you practice today and this week?
- What activities do you need to stop or reduce? How will you implement those changes today and this week?
- How can you work to ensure you're giving energy and attention to solving activities each day?
- What will solving look like for you today?
- How will you demonstrate creative, energetic problem-solving?

PART TWO

Creating the Change You Crave

TEN

Value Your Questions over Answers

"I do not fix problems. I fix my thinking then the problems fix themselves."

—LOUISE HAY

Questions are one of the most effective tools you can use in your quest to become a better thinker. Better thinkers are better problem solvers. As you become a better problem solver, you become an increasingly capable change agent in *every* area of your life. In times when you feel stuck or feel convinced that you *can't* change how you think or act, questions are a powerful, free tool.

Questions unlock new possibilities while drawing you out of your past patterns. Use them and use them often, because your questions are worth *far* more than your answers.

Think for a minute about how often you negotiate with yourself. You reopen cases you've already closed in order to justify what you want now. You argue in favor of an excuse. You hold yourself back by building a case *against* what you want most, in favor of what's more appealing in the moment. You let emotions cloud your perspective and you give those emotions a vote in the choices you make.

Building a practice of asking yourself questions will help you see the flaws in your excuses, stop negotiating for delay, and minimize the frequency of emotionally driven decisions.

Questions help you resolve internal debates with the best choices, not just the easiest, most familiar, or most convenient ones.

With better questions, asked more frequently and answered more honestly, you'll begin to **take away the power you've been giving to all those self-limiting beliefs** because new options will immediately become both clearer and more compelling.

Questions will help you challenge the beliefs that are currently limiting your potential and your progress.

Instead of defaulting to "I'm an emotional eater" as a justification for a night of chocolate and wine, questions open up the potential for other options.

What else could I be? What other choices could I make tonight? Am I capable of choosing something else just for today? Do I want to continue to endorse that belief? How do I feel when I make that choice? What choices would I have to make tonight in order to wake up feeling great tomorrow?

When good questions are answered honestly, the "should I or shouldn't I?" debate becomes more balanced. It becomes more honest and less biased toward habit, history, drama, emotion, temptation, and preference.

Instead of getting locked in on making a case for why you *should* watch another episode before bed or why you *should* have the bread from the breadbasket the waiter just placed in front of you, questions prompt you to also consider the other side of the coin—why you *shouldn't* make those choices.

Whether you're aware of it or not, you automatically ask and answer hundreds, if not thousands, of questions each day without ever verbalizing them.

Consider thoughts like:

Oh! I really want those shoes!

I'm dying for something sweet!

I really don't want to get up and go to the gym. I want to sleep a little longer.

With those thoughts, you're looking to give yourself permission. You're trying to make a case for what you want, or want to avoid. These are actually implied questions.

Should I buy those shoes?

Can I have this dessert?

Will I hit snooze and skip today's workout?

Your thoughts are the answer and the process by which you convince yourself of every choice you make.

"The first principle is that you must not fool yourself and you are the easiest person to fool."

—RICHARD FEYNMAN

Ah, how brilliantly we can fool ourselves!

One of my clients is a lawyer. She's brilliant and tenacious. She's a great debater, which undoubtedly makes her a great attorney, but she uses those skills against herself. She can make a case that justifies *any* choice. She'll not only give herself permission to overindulge, she can effectively convince herself that it's a good idea!

One afternoon I asked her if she noticed that she has a pattern of making the same decision over and over again.

She'll decide that she isn't going to drink alcohol this week. The following day, though the decision has already been made and the case is closed, she'll reopen it. *Should I drink today? Maybe just one glass of wine at the cocktail party? Hey, it's better than I used to do! As long as I eat really clean, or maybe if I fast, it won't hurt. There's no harm in one glass of wine.* The following day, she'll participate in the same internal debate, considering once again if she should drink.

This is an exhausting way to live and a real threat to consistency. Every single day she is capable of convincing herself to drink. Every single day she is *also* capable of convincing herself *not* to drink. It boils down to the way she *chooses* to think. I challenged her to use the power of questions to break the habit of deciding on the same issue over and over and over again.

The simple question I suggested is "Have I already decided on this issue?"

The question serves as a pattern interrupt. She's already proven that she can convince herself that a drink is deserved or that it won't thwart her goals. Asking this question reminds her that she doesn't need to exhaust herself in this way. She doesn't need to participate in the daily debate. The case is closed. It also helps her avoid continuing to erode her trust in the decisions she makes.

Have I already decided on this issue?

Yes. I'm not drinking this week.

No further thoughts needed on this topic at this time.

We are all brilliant and skilled at negotiating with ourselves. We fool ourselves most easily because we know what works! As rational creatures, we can justify just about any choice in the world.

Want chips? You can make a case for it.

Want to skip your workout? You can make a case for it.

Want to charge that cute shirt to your credit card? You can make a case for it.

Want to binge? You can talk yourself into it and even convince yourself that it's a *good* idea!

Just because you can defend the choice doesn't make it true, right, or best. Author Stephen King summarizes this as only a great writer can: "the answer isn't always the truth."

We talk ourselves into what we want in a moment, even when the logic we use isn't true and the choices we're defending don't serve our goals. We can justify choices that hurt us, make us sick, and hold us back. It's remarkable, really, and questions will help you step away from that broken pattern so you can stop living so small (and making yourself so crazy).

There are some nuances to this strategy, however, because sometimes the logic you use to justify an excuse or exception is *actually* true. Sometimes the questions you ask will support the choices that derail your goals.

For example: you're trying to stay on budget but find yourself making a case for a new pair of shoes.

You ask yourself, "Do I really want them?"

Yes!

Or you're stressed about a big work project and you want a glass of wine after dinner.

You ask yourself, "Will this help me unwind?"

Yes!

Okay, now what?

One of the primary reasons most people are inconsistent is that their excuses are in fact true or, at a minimum, *believed* to be true. In fact, the most dangerous excuses *are* true.

Through questions, you'll learn to challenge your view of reality and evaluate if something else is *more* true. You begin to see more clearly how, when focusing on one small truth, you overlook the complete picture of the truth.

I don't watch a lot of television, but I'm a fan of the Showtime original *Billions*. If you haven't seen it, it's about money and power within a successful hedge fund. The company has an in-house psychiatrist, Wendy, whose job it is to make sure all the traders stay mentally sharp.

In one of the early episodes of season two, the firm bets against a space mission and ends up making a tremendous profit when the mission fails and everyone onboard the spacecraft dies. Taylor, an executive at the center of the controversial gamble, is struggling with the fact that the firm profited from such a tragedy. Taylor meets with Wendy to get some advice and work through the conflict of values.

Wendy reminds Taylor that in life, things will always be in conflict and there will always be multiple versions of the truth. But, she advises him, **"When you're here, mind the truth that makes you money."**

Like Taylor, you'll find yourself facing conflicting truths every single day.

You want ice cream—true.

You want to lose weight—also true.

Mind the truth that moves you forward.

Mind the truth that supports your goals.

Mind the truth that creates the change you crave.

You want that new pair of shoes—true.

You want to get out of debt—also true.

Mind the truth that moves you forward.

Mind the truth that supports your goals.

Mind the truth that creates the change you crave.

Your husband didn't follow through on his word and you're mad—true.

You value a strong marriage over proving a point and being passive-aggressive—also true.

Mind the truth that moves you forward.

Mind the truth that supports your goals.

Mind the truth that creates the change you crave.

As you begin to make a decision, you might initially see only the **emotional corner of truth** that justifies what you want in that moment. Pause to ask and answer: *What is the truth that moves me forward?*

Asking questions will slow you down just enough to break free from the grips of past patterns so you can evaluate the complete truth and the version of it that takes you where you want to go, instead of the version that keeps you from it.

Good questions, answered honestly, help you challenge the accuracy and completeness of your thinking. When you are willing to ask yourself questions and challenge what you believe to be true, you can completely reframe your thinking.

A client recently told me that she binged on cookies, despite wanting to lose weight. Prior to the binge, she was feeling stressed about work and thought, *Who cares? Why do I even try?*

There's always a thought or series of thoughts that precede your choices. Questions allow you to identify and challenge them.

In that moment, she certainly felt like *Who cares?* was a real, valid, and true thought. It was certainly a piece of the truth and a perspective that would effectively talk her into what she wanted in that moment: cookies. Here's the thing: it's not the **complete** truth. It's an emotional corner of the truth that serves the feeling of the moment and not the full reality of her capabilities or goals.

Without a doubt, those kinds of thoughts can be a barrier to creating change. You can *know* what to do, but if you convince yourself that it's true that you don't care, you won't act on what you know.

It's like you put blinders on, obscuring from your view the many other relevant factors like why you *do* care, how you'll feel after binging, and if the cookies are a worthwhile trade for your goals and progress.

By asking a better set of questions, she was able to challenge that story and step into the whole truth. Questions help you break the unconscious habit of thinking in incomplete thoughts and ideas so you can respond to the whole truth.

Before getting to the better set of questions, however, my client and I had to acknowledge the question she asked herself: *Who cares?*

I'm sure you've played that card, too.

Stop acting as though that's a rhetorical question. And just so we're all on the same page, let's define "rhetorical question."

The Merriam-Webster Dictionary defines rhetorical question as a question not intended to require an answer.

Who cares? cannot be rhetorical in your life any longer. It *does* require an answer.

The next time you ask yourself "who cares" about your choice, your goal, your actions, or your progress, answer the question. Who *does* care?

I prefer this definition of rhetorical question from Dictionary.com:

"A question asked in order to create a dramatic effect or to make a point rather than to get an answer."

Okay, the point has been made and the drama won't serve you. The next time you ask yourself questions like "Who cares? Why do I even try? What's the point?" remind yourself that these are not rhetorical. You will answer them. The answer matters.

If you're going to use a question in your argument or rationalization, for Pete's sake, you owe yourself an answer. It's simply not fair to use questions in the process of excuse-making but fail to answer them. You can do better. It's time to be a more mature thinker.

Without an answer, the permissive question isn't real; it's just a card you play to let yourself off the hook. It's not an actual feeling or thought; it's the "Get Out of Jail Free" card you've stacked in your deck. Only you can decide if you will keep that card in your deck of options or set it aside and take it out of play in your life.

What are some of the permissive questions or statements you use to justify choices that aren't aligned with your goals?

"I define myself more by my questions than by my answers."

—ELIE WIESEL

Questions will help you counteract your fears and doubts as you challenge your assumptions, judgments, and insecurities. When you face them head on, you can control them instead of allowing them to subtly and continuously control you.

Recently, I got an email from a client who expressed that she was at the end of her rope. I could sense the defeat in her email. "If I can't be successful at the thing I want the most, then there's no hope. It can't happen."

She explained that the thing she wanted *most* in the world was to lose weight, but even with that burning desire, she wasn't doing the work. She was still overeating and overindulging on a regular basis.

I listened patiently and responded with a few questions for her to consider.

"You're telling me that you want to lose weight more than anything in the world. Do you want to lose weight more than you want to overeat? Do your patterns of behavior reflect that? Is that true in your mind or is it true in your actions? If it's in fact true that you want to lose weight more than anything in the world, are you reminding yourself of that as you consider your choices in a moment of temptation?"

She was initially defensive. It's not comfortable to admit that your choices don't match what you say you want—especially when it's something you want badly. That's a hard thing for anyone to acknowledge. However, using questions to get to the complete version of the truth is empowering. It moves you away from being a victim and feeling powerless to realizing that you hold all the power and the solution is much closer than you think.

When your questions poke holes in your problems, it's not about criticism or judgment; **it's simply an opportunity for an honest assessment of what is really happening in _action_ versus what is happening in _thoughts_.** It's an opportunity to assess whether or not your intentions align with your actions.

Not only were this client's actions and intentions not aligned, they were in direct opposition.

Think about all the times you've been discouraged. That discouragement comes when you aren't viewing the totality of the situation or acknowledging your innate power to change it. You're fixed on the problem.

Questions eliminate the drama, story, and victimization.

DECIDING UNDER THE INFLUENCE (DUI)

I want to help you bring awareness and improvement to a huge barrier to change that also strips so much joy from life: DUI, or deciding under the influence.

I'm pretty sure you can relate to this one. Deciding under the influence of emotion, deciding under the influence of stress, deciding under the influence of drama...it doesn't lead to your best decisions.

This *doesn't* mean that we avoid making decisions when life gets tough. Every single one of us has to make decisions when life feels easy as well as when it feels hard. What you need to practice is using questions to break through the filter of stress, emotion, or fatigue so you can consistently make rational, healthy decisions.

I remind myself of this practice with a simple phrase.

Don't draw conclusions from illusions. Don't believe everything you think and don't believe everything you feel.

Questions are the tool that will make you less likely to jump to conclusions and help you slow down enough to make a great decision and have a measured response. Questions can help protect you from emotional reactions and return you to a place of control.

Once, after seriously dating a guy for a little over a year, he told me he wasn't in love with me. For quite some time we had been saying "I love you," and one evening I playfully asked, "Are you in love with me?" and he casually replied, "I don't know."

It wasn't what I expected him to say and my emotional brain seemed to instantaneously replace my logical brain. I felt gut-punched.

I started to cry. Though he said, "I don't know," I heard "no."

Quite different, right? I was, out of habit, drawing conclusions from illusions. **I got lost in what I heard instead of staying connected to what was actually said.** I allowed my fear to create a version of reality that was true to me but certainly wasn't *the* truth. I was officially under the influence of emotion. Danger zone.

Not one to backpedal, he matter-of-factly explained that he didn't really know the difference between loving someone and being *in* love. He didn't think he had ever been in love before and acknowledged that there were moments where he felt like he was *in* love with me, but he couldn't be sure since he wasn't able to define what "in love" means.

He asked *me* what I thought it meant to be in love and I had to admit I wasn't sure how to define it either.

Though I could see his point, our evening ended abruptly. I was emotional. I was making assumptions and I just didn't want him around.

Throughout the night, my brain twisted wildly with fears and worry. *He doesn't love me. He doesn't want to be with me. We're over. I deserve better.*

Drama.

Drama stems from what we add to the facts. We create drama (as I did in this situation) anytime we lean on our own interpretation instead of staying connected to what *actually* happened. Drama is introduced when we make assumptions and jump to conclusions.

I used questions to force myself to slow down and lift the veil of emotion so I could make better decisions. These questions also helped me avoid unnecessary negative emotion. I started by asking some simple questions I use often.

What *actually* happened?

What's the difference between what actually happened and my feelings about what happened?

What's the difference between what actually happened and what I'm telling myself happened?

What else might this mean?

I wanted to consider all the options instead of clinging to my first, most emotional conclusion.

- He *is* in love with me but doesn't know how to define it.
- He's not in love with me and it doesn't matter. He still wants to be with me.
- He's not in love with me and doesn't want to be with me. (This is purely speculation and not what he said.)
- He values telling me what is real over telling me what he thinks I want to hear. I like that. In fact, I encourage that in him.

I turned to more questions and, with each one, I developed a more complete version of the truth, dialed back my emotion, felt less upset, and identified where I was straight-up inventing things that never happened. **Instead of staying in my emotion and fueling my feelings with attention, I chose to question my answers, challenge my assumptions, and differentiate between reality and my mental inventions.** With each question, I moved further from past patterns and drama, and closer to the complete truth. I also quickly calmed myself down.

Here are some helpful questions I use when I find myself under the influence of emotion.

- What meaning have I attached to the situation?
- Is that true?
- What else could it mean?
- What emotions might be clouding my reaction?
- What is happening without my story about what's happening?

These questions are powerful, not just in relationships but also in your work and your own choices. Using them will help you see and experience that the **drama and emotion is often optional and invented.** If you can't recognize it and don't practice separating yourself from the drama, it can defeat you and drain your energy. Drama is emotional waste.

(Funny side note: the next day, we asked his mom how she would describe the difference between loving someone and being in love. She said, "When you're in love, you just know you can't live without the other person." I put my hand on his arm, shrugged, and said, "You're off the hook, babe. If that's what it is, I'm not in love with you either." We all laughed. I could certainly live without him, and he without me.)

The next time you get an email you interpret as rude or you have an interaction where you think someone is being dismissive, break your pattern of assumption and resist the temptation to respond to your initial interpretation by asking, "What else could this mean?"

There are things, right now, that you staunchly believe about yourself, your goals, and the barriers keeping you from achieving them that are *completely untrue*. There are things you believe about people in your life and interactions you've had that are just as untrue. These beliefs just haven't been challenged and clarified. Whether you know it yet or not, you've drawn many wrong conclusions from many emotional or habitual illusions.

Questions will set you free. Because the choices you make are significantly influenced by how you feel, **using questions to deliver yourself to emotional sobriety is a play for the front of your life's playbook.**

BUILDING A HABIT OF QUESTIONS

A couple years ago, while I was preparing for ASCEND, a Primal Potential weekend workshop, I invited my mom and sister out to dinner. I wanted to try out an activity in advance of the event and they were about to be my guinea pigs.

I explained that I wanted to do a workshop at the event where we **exclusively communicate with questions.**

No statements or explanations, only questions. Everything must be spoken as inquiry.

The purpose of the activity would be to get everyone focused on solutions instead of defending their behavior or making a case for the validity of the problem.

That's a common pattern when problem-solving. We *love* to explain the problem and then substantiate it. We explain the circumstances and justify why the problem exists. Often, instead of trying to identify and implement potential solutions, we merely build a case for the problem.

When we're sharing problems with others, it often becomes a tug-of-war of opinions and perspectives and we're more concerned with being right than getting it right.

Questions will require that you set aside your ego. They shift your focus from what or who is right and help you figure out how to **make** it right. When you're questioning, you aren't defending or justifying. Defending and justifying do not help you create change—they're behaviors connected to problems, not to solutions.

This questions-only activity would hopefully break through a challenge or obstacle by **employing curiosity and avoid-**

ing defensiveness. I asked my mom and sister which of them would be willing to share a problem, in the form of a question, to kick off our little dinnertime experiment.

I was surprised when my sister asked, "How do I balance getting out of debt and enjoying my life?"

Years earlier she and I had pledged to *stop* talking to each other about money. Money had always been a struggle for Debi. We approached finances differently. I am a saver. She was a spender. We had countless discussions about her financial situation and they never ended well. I'd tell her what to do; she'd tell me why she couldn't do it that way. We'd both get frustrated, righteous, and defensive.

Yet here she was, offering it up as the subject of this exercise. I think my mom wanted to escape to the ladies' room. This topic usually led to hurt feelings, followed by awkward silence.

I took a deep breath and dove into the next question.

I asked, "Do you think it has to be one or the other?"

"What if it does?"

I decided to start with the most basic thing, "What are the ways to have more money?"

She asked, "What are they?"

"What can you do other than make more money?"

"What?"

My mom and I exchanged glances. Does Debi *really* not know that the other option is spending less? Fortunately, my goal here was *not* to be condescending.

Though habit was tempting me to sigh and respond, "Seriously?" (hey, fair game, it is a question) I asked, "Can you spend less money?"

This is where things would normally get dicey and defensive.

She answered honestly, "What if I don't want to spend less money?"

We used questions to get closer to the truth instead of using justifications to move further from it.

I asked her, "Are you really enjoying your life with the financial stress you have right now? Is this the way you want things to be? It seems like you don't want to spend less because you associate spending more with enjoying your life more? But are you really enjoying life right now?

Might it be possible that spending less would actually allow you to enjoy life more?"

She sat quietly.

She was considering, open-mindedly this time, that maybe spending *less* would allow her to actually enjoy life *more*, not the other way around. There was something more true than the story she had been clinging to about her spending.

Spending money was actually limiting her. It was creating stress in her life, not removing it. It was making her life smaller, not bigger.

Since that conversation, Debi's finances have undoubtedly transformed. She's created changes that allow her to both make more money and spend less. She has opened up a private practice, asked for and received a raise at her job, and paid off all her credit cards. The discipline she brings to her financial choices has allowed her to enjoy life more, not less, because she's gradually eliminating one of her biggest stressors: money problems.

That short exercise was a starting point—it represented a shift in the way she was willing to think about money and her ability to create change.

That's always the most important step. As Louise Hay

reminded us at the top of the chapter, when you fix your thinking, your problems fix themselves!

Even beyond the financial considerations, this questions-only exercise was powerful for both of us, as it was the first time we were able to talk about money without becoming defensive and judgmental. We used questions to focus on opening up and exploring options without letting defenses get in the way.

The questions themselves didn't create results for Debi and they won't for you, either. In fact, someone recently asked me if questions just keep you spinning your wheels in a place of thought instead of action.

No. They absolutely don't. Great questions are a critical precursor to effective action. The right questions focus you on the steps you can take to create your solution. The right questions clear out initial emotional filters and illuminate incorrect assumptions so the action you take has the intended effect. If your questions don't lead you to improved action, you aren't asking the right questions.

The right questions aren't focused on problems or obstacles. They aren't focused on future challenges or fears or even future strategies. They snap you right out of the tendency to fixate on the past. The right questions point you squarely to what you can and will do right now to create change today.

There's a big difference between "I want to lose weight" or "I want to make more money" (intention without action) and "What will I do today to make it happen? What is a choice I can make right now that will move me in that direction?" (attention on action).

"Genius is in the idea. Impact, however, comes from action."

—SIMON SINEK

WHAT TO DO WHEN YOU DON'T KNOW

What do you do when you don't *know* the answer to your question?

We often dismiss questions by saying "I don't know" or "I'm confused" to avoid taking ownership of our role in a solution and delay doing work.

As I see it, those responses are cop-outs. You don't have to know the answer, but let's acknowledge the fact that you are capable of *finding* it.

"I don't know" might mean "I haven't done the work yet" or "I need to ask more questions here" or "I need to take some action or do some work to get clearer on an answer or solution."

Sit with it. Ask yourself, "How can I find the answer?" or "What might be the answer? What are some options?"

You can absolutely find your answers. Questions help you navigate to answers.

Confusion is the beginning of understanding, not the end.

Knowledge is not a prerequisite for action. Knowledge is an end result of action.

If you aren't sure of an answer, take action. Do something. You'll learn from what you try. Stop holding yourself back from action because you're waiting for answers. Create the answers. They are waiting for you on the other side of intelligent action.

Don't wait to think up a solution. Create it. Travel to it. Your solutions are in your progress and attention. You will always learn more from action than from thought. When you aren't sure, start seeking answers through your own practice.

BECOME YOUR OWN CLEARNESS COMMITTEE

I wish I could take credit for the idea of a "clearness committee"—I love it and think it's another way to use this tool of questioning. The concept of a clearness committee actually dates all the way back to the 1600s.

The Quakers developed these clearness committees to help community members solve problems via this **question-based process of discernment.**

When I read that, the first thing I did was look up the actual definition of the word "discernment": **the ability to judge well.**

Clearness committees would generate questions when someone needed to gain clarity and develop the ability to judge well and think beyond his or her initial perceptions.

That's exactly why we're learning to use questions! So we can develop the ability to judge well and go beyond our initial perceptions.

We all have the ability to use questions in moments of decision-making to slow down, go beyond perception, and develop the skill of judging well.

In fact, we all need to do this more often. I'd argue for

holding your own personal clearness committee every day!

You can probably think about particular recurring moments when you could benefit from a personal clearness committee. Maybe when you're beating yourself up for a choice you wish you hadn't made or when you're worked up after a tense staff meeting.

What would it look like to take three minutes to hold your own personal clearness committee? Or is there someone in your life with whom you could call these mini-sessions as needed? In these sessions, use questions—either ones from this chapter or ones you develop on your own—to improve your ability to judge the situation well.

You can start with one simple question, like "What's the difference between what actually happened and how I feel about what happened?"

Or you can try something a little more structured, like the process suggested by author Katherine Rosback. She encourages a strategy she calls 4-24: setting aside four minutes every twenty-four hours to practice asking better questions.

What if you built this in as a part of your morning routine?

Or in response to temptation or frustration? Four minutes of questions.

You don't need to answer the questions in this four-minute block; just brainstorm questions about your goals, actions, emotions, situations, circumstances, or perspectives.

Create clarity and inform intelligent action through questions.

CREATE CHANGE CHALLENGE

In your next moment of temptation or emotion, set your timer for four minutes and ask yourself questions until time expires. It's not a race to see how many questions you can generate. Be thoughtful. Think differently. Explore all your options and consider what else is true. For this challenge, the key is to write all the questions down on paper. You recruit more brainpower when you write ideas down than when merely thinking about them.

ELEVEN

Simplicity

"Somewhere along the way in your life, you became unwilling to take baby steps. You lost faith in the universal truth that the simplest little disciplines done again and again over time would move the mightiest mountains."

—JEFF OLSON

Most of us love the *idea* of working *with* ourselves instead of *against* ourselves, but don't know how to *do* it. We can agree that working with ourselves *sounds* easier than the alternative, but aren't clear on how to turn this concept into a daily practice and personal operating system.

If I could capture it in a word, the word would be "**simplicity.**" Making change easier requires that you pursue simplicity in your thoughts and in your actions.

Though it's normal to be drawn to the complex and complicated, the easiest, most effective path is usually the simplest one. The intricate plan is often appealing and exciting, but rarely sustainable. After all, **complexity is the enemy of execution.**

One of the most obvious outward examples of the contrast between complex and simple can be seen in every fitness center. If you've ever been in a gym, you've not only seen this play out, you've probably been one of these two types of people.

In every gym you'll notice the wanderers. They have great intentions, but they're *all over* the place. They are not focused or efficient. They wander from machine to machine, casually giving it a whirl, often spending more time trying to figure out how it works than actually *using* it. They're aimless, easily distracted, and not getting in a great workout. They fiddle with their music, take frequent water breaks, check their phone, and chat with anyone who makes eye contact.

Sure, the wanderer showed up, but their energy and effort aren't driving much in terms of results. Their approach is not focused, simple, or effective.

The other group *is* focused. They go into the gym with a purpose. They don't want to chat. They keep to themselves—their heads are down and their music is up. They know what they are there to do and they get it done. They're efficient. They spend less time, spend less mental and emotional energy, and get better results.

These two groups in the gym represent the two paths to change. You can be whirling around, incredibly busy, trying out a little bit of everything, but not really getting where you want to go. With that approach, every day has significant variation in terms of effort, motivation, and focus.

Or you can be focused. You can choose to pursue simplicity by refusing to indulge distractions that keep you from the life you want.

I think you can probably see that one of the primary reasons the hard road is so dang hard is that **we're inefficient, inconsistent, distracted, trying out every possible option, and grabbing up every excuse that presents itself.**

The easier road is shorter, straighter, and far more effective. Choosing a practice of pursuing simplicity will undeniably make change (and life) easier.

The simple path to change can be summarized with one of my favorite mantras. In the form of a question, it offers both simplification and marching orders:

What can I release that is no longer serving me?

Yes, it's simple. It's also powerful. Too often, we dismiss chances to change because we think they are too simple—too simple to make a difference. We convince ourselves that it's "not enough," even when it's more than you could ever need, if you would only do something with it!

We'll look at specific strategies for embracing simplicity, but before we do, we have to break down this major barrier to change—dismissing things that are simple and straightforward.

PENNIES AND INCHES

Have you heard of the paradox of the growing heap? It poses a theoretical question: If you pour a bag of rice on the table, and then move just one grain of rice to the other side of the table, how many heaps do you have? One or two? You can hardly call one grain of rice a heap, right? What if you move two or three grains of rice to join the solitary one? At what point does the smaller pile become a heap?

This paradox reminds us that no single grain of rice, or no single action, can be easily identified as the one that made the difference. Yet, at some point, one single grain *has* to be the one that made the difference.

There is a tipping point, and it is reached by just one grain of rice.

You might also see this paradox described with money. If ten coins aren't enough to make a man rich, what if you add one? Inevitably, you'll arrive at a point where you'll have to conclude that one single coin made the difference.

This paradox is at play in our own lives every day. One workout doesn't make a person fit, right? But what happens when one becomes two, two becomes three, and we progress into the hundreds? At what point is a person fit?

One indulgence doesn't make a person overweight, right? But what happens when one becomes two, two becomes three, or three becomes four?

You inevitably reach a point where *one* made the difference.

The smallest, simplest things we're likely to dismiss are the very things that create change. They are not, in fact, too small to make a difference—they are actually the difference maker!

This perspective has always felt powerful for me, and it played a role in the mindset shift that transformed my whole life. I used to throw away pennies. If I was cleaning out my car and there were a few pennies on the floorboard, I'd vacuum them up. If I was emptying out a purse and there were some dirty pennies at the bottom, I'd throw them in the trash. I told myself that pennies were worthless. Sure, they are money, but I thought they weren't enough to make a difference.

That's categorically untrue. I'm telling you this because I didn't have a penny problem; I had a perspective problem.

It wasn't just that I didn't value small amounts of money, I didn't value *anything* small. It wasn't just pennies I dismissed as too small to make a difference—I'd tell myself to go ahead and have dessert because skipping this one brownie wouldn't make a difference anyway. I'd hit the snooze button on my alarm clock because cutting my morning ten minutes short wouldn't matter. I'd avoid working out when I only had twenty minutes because that length of a workout was too short to make a difference anyway.

That perspective made change infinitely harder. It created a no-win scenario.

The small things I *could* do were too small to bother with, but at the same time, I'd look at big changes as things I *couldn't* do or wasn't ready for.

What a pickle—the small things are too small and the big things are too big.

If you added up all the changes I dismissed because I told myself they were too small to make a difference, I could have transformed my life twenty times over by now.

The problem wasn't with the pennies. The problem was my mental operating system of dismissing the small things as worthless.

I can't pinpoint when this thinking shifted for me, but at some point, I started literally picking up pennies wherever I found them—in the grocery store, on the sidewalk, everywhere. I started to get really excited about pennies! I'd go out of my way to grab them!

One day I was walking with my mom and I stopped to pick up a dirty penny on a sidewalk. "That's gross!" she said. "Leave it there!"

I stopped, picked it up, and tucked it in my pocket.

There is no minimum threshold that needs to be met for money to have value to me. I simply value money.

Similarly, there's no improvement that is too small to matter. There is no minimum threshold of time, effort, or impact that must be met for an action or thought to have value.

Value the good choices that are teeny and the good choices that are big. They all matter. Besides, the teeny ones are easier and available more frequently.

It's about seeing and seizing opportunities of all sizes.

Where do you dismiss choices as too small to make a difference? What else might be true?

One of my favorite movies is *Any Given Sunday*—a football movie starring one of my favorite actors, Al Pacino. There's a scene in the movie that has become a viral sensation online since its 1999 release. Pacino, who coaches the team, is giving his young players a passionate locker-room speech at halftime. The team is down and they haven't been playing with heart. He tells his players that life and football are both games of inches. They're won and lost by inches, and if you want to win, you have to fight for the inches.

He tells his team, "The inches we need are everywhere around us! They are in every break of the game. Every minute, every second. On this team, we fight for that inch!"

Friend, the inches you need are all around you. They are

in every moment of your day. They are in every choice you make. If you want to win, you have to fight for the inches—they make or break the game. They are certainly *not* too small to matter. They matter most.

This is a perspective change that requires *practice*. You have to train yourself *out* of the pattern of dismissing a workout as too short to matter or a bite of food as too small to make a difference. You have to work to reframe the idea that one day isn't enough to move the needle.

The little things are the big things. It's not that the small choice will make or break your journey, but the mental operating system of either embracing or dismissing the small things will.

If you can do ten bodyweight squats while you brush your teeth, it matters.

If you can save one dollar today, it matters.

If you can pass up the small piece of candy you usually grab from the candy bowl at work, it matters.

Nothing is too small to move the needle. These choices are small and they are simple. They are easy to do, but they're just as easy not to do. This is where you need to practice.

In his book *The Slight Edge*, author Jeff Olson makes this case for the power of the small, simple choices. He writes, "Somewhere along the way in your life, you became unwilling to take baby steps. You lost faith in the universal truth that the simple little disciplines done again and again over time would move the mightiest mountains."

Little disciplines, done again and again over time will move the mightiest mountains.

Isn't that so encouraging? Remember we said at the start of this book that change is created through evolution, not revolution.

You don't need to begin with a 180-degree change in your behavior. You begin with small, simple daily disciplines and you return to your practice each day.

Use the power of questions to lead you from this idea into your own practice:

What simple daily discipline will you execute today?

To further demonstrate this point of simplicity, Olson goes on to explain the compounding power of a penny.

When given the choice between one million dollars or the sum of one single penny doubled every day for one month, most people choose the million dollars. They certainly would *not* make that choice if they realized that a penny, doubled every day for **just one month**, adds up to nearly eleven million dollars. One month. Pennies. Eleven million dollars.

This is why you can't continue to dismiss the power of the small, simple steps.

Think for a second about financial investing. The tenets of successful investing are quite simple.

Start small.

Start now.

Be consistent.

Small is big over time.

Be patient.

What if that were your mental operating system as you went through each day? What would that look like?

Start small.

Start now.

Be consistent.

Small is big over time.

Be patient.

If this were your operating system today, what would it look like? How are you able and willing to put this into practice today?

What are those super simple thoughts, actions, or choices that are always lying around, that you've previously thought as too small to make a difference? Grab them up. They add up quickly. The inches are all around you.

Success isn't about doing four thousand things. It's about doing **simple things** four thousand times.

Change is created when you commit to executing ridiculously simple strategies made of ridiculously simple actions.

Master the mundane and refuse to overlook simplicity.

Little hinges swing big doors.

These simple daily disciplines will take you into what is called the cycle of accelerated returns. Instead of trying to motivate yourself to take some big step or execute a long-term strategy, pursue the simplest possible step you can make **today.**

As you make these simple choices that feel almost too small to matter, you'll build both confidence and momentum. With increasing confidence and momentum, you'll be drawn toward more of those small, simple choices and you'll see results. Change and progress will feel easier. As you do more, you'll see more results, which will fuel more positive feelings and therefore more action. Use simplicity to throw yourself into that cycle of accelerated returns.

THINKING SIMPLY

We obstruct the process of change and needlessly overwhelm ourselves when we complicate our decision-making process. By adding in emotional considerations, the weight of past patterns, and concerns about the future, we make change so much harder than it needs to be.

There are two things that don't need to factor into your decision-making:

1. The past
2. The future

Your ability to change isn't defined by yesterday and doesn't have anything to do with what happens tomorrow.

A few months back, I shared a personal challenge I gave myself while traveling to a conference. I spent a week in San Diego and I wanted to feel really great about my choices instead of using travel to justify eating too much, drinking too much, and spending too much money.

For most of my life, traveling was one of many circumstances I'd use to add unnecessary complexity to my decision-making process. Instead of keeping things simple and straightforward, I'd make a case for how strict I'd be when I returned home or how I'd get all the junk food out of my system so I'd be ready to rein things in after a couple of days.

Never true. I wasn't thinking simply.

On this particular trip to the West Coast, I decided to try a new, simple strategy.

My challenge to myself was to be completely myopic in every decision I made.

Basically, I was putting my blinders on. As I made every choice—if I should work out, what workout I should do, when I should eat, what I should eat, etc.—I only considered what was my best *in that moment*.

That was it. No past. No future. No story. No debate. No negotiation. No justification. No promises for what would come after.

I refused to consider past factors, like "Well, I've been really good today, so..." or "I had such a hard workout earlier, therefore..."

Similarly, I wouldn't consider how strict I'd be tomorrow, what I'd eat later on, or how I might work out that evening. Nope, that doesn't have *anything* to do with what's in front of me right now. Just now. What is my best in *this* moment?

The practice reminded me of a quote from Navy SEAL commander and author of *Discipline Equals Freedom*, Jocko Willink.

"You have to decide that you are going to be in control, that you are going to do what YOU want to do. Weakness doesn't get a vote. Laziness doesn't get a vote. Sadness doesn't get a vote. Frustration doesn't get a vote. NEGATIVITY doesn't get a vote."

In my case, the past didn't get a vote. Tomorrow didn't

get a vote. My energy level, emotions, stress, frustration, geographical location—they didn't get a vote. The only vote was from the simple question, asked repeatedly:

What is my *best* choice in *this* moment?

Bringing in the past ("It's so much better than I used to do") or the future ("I'll be better tomorrow") is a **red flag.** You're negotiating. You're justifying. And **that's only something we do when we're trying to make something okay, that, when looked at on its own, isn't in our best interests.** You're choosing complexity over simplicity.

When you find that you are talking yourself into having a cookie because you haven't eaten much today, you're bringing the past into a present-moment decision. The past doesn't get a vote.

Practice keeping it simple: Is this your best choice in this moment?

When you find yourself justifying a second drink because you won't drink tomorrow, you're bringing the future into a present-moment decision. The future doesn't get a vote.

Return to the simple mantra I shared at the start of the chapter: What can I release that is no longer serving me?

Maybe that inquiring reminds you to stop scrolling through Facebook so you can finish your work, or maybe it encourages you to avoid sugar tonight.

Now demands your best and simplicity is always available to you. There's nothing about yesterday or tomorrow, earlier or later, that needs to factor into what you choose now and next.

SIMPLICITY IN PROBLEM-SOLVING

The next time you find yourself wound tight or overwhelmed by a problem or challenge, practice returning to simplicity. Yes, you can layer on complexity by running in circles around the problem like the wanderer at the gym. You can stay in your emotions, complain, and convince yourself that you're a victim. Or you can give your energy to the simplest version of the solution.

Here's a practice I find super helpful when I have a chance to practice solving problems more simply:

Define the problem in one sentence.

You're not alone if you initially find this hard. Most of us have deeply engrained patterns of wanting to explain or justify the problem and include all sorts of information about how it makes us feel. Practice your way out of the habit.

Stick to simplicity and define it in just one sentence.

From there, give your energy to the solution. Practice the customer service approach we explored in Part One and begin to creatively and energetically explore all your options for a solution.

Then, take action!

Resist the common approach of talking for hours, weeks, or even years about the problem.

I complained about my job for years. I complained about the people I worked for, the way they made decisions, the way they communicated, and their priorities. I complained about the workload and staffing. I complained about unrealistic deadlines and people who ignored the facts. Honestly, I complained about this every single day for years.

I cringe when I think about the poor people in my life who had to listen to my whining, complaining, and negativity for so long.

If someone had said to me, "In one sentence, what is the

problem?" I would have said, "I can't stand the environment in which I work."

If only they had then said, "Great. Stop complaining and get to work on a solution."

I so wish I had such a breath of fresh air in my life at the time. Now I get to be that breath of fresh air for you.

It might be that you're addicted to the problem, but I'm telling you—if you want a solution, there's a simple one waiting for you. The inches are all around you!

CREATE CHANGE CHALLENGE

Decide on a twenty-four-hour period within the next week when you will practice living by simple decision-making criteria. You can choose the challenge I gave myself, where you simply make your best choice in every moment, without negotiation or debate. Or maybe your simple decision-making criterion is that you only talk about solutions. That means for twenty-four hours there's no complaining, gossiping, or worrying, as none of those behaviors are related to solutions. Recruit a friend or family member and see what a difference a day can make!

What simple decision-making criteria will you employ for your twenty-four-hour challenge?

TWELVE

Become a Solution Person

"Out beyond ideas of wrongdoing and right doing there is a field.

I'll meet you there."

—RUMI

I've heard it said that if you share a problem more than twice without taking action to fix it, you aren't looking for a solution, you're looking for attention.

That stings a little, right? **It stings because it's true.**

In our attempts to create change, we give too much energy to the problems in our lives and not nearly enough energy to creating solutions.

Though it can be uncomfortable to admit when you're doing this—it pokes at your ego—the awareness of the pattern gives you an opportunity to make change easier.

Remember back in Part One where we talked about customer service being an inside job? We explored the way staying in the sensing part of the problem keeps us from moving into solving mode.

In this chapter, we will explore strategies and tools for noticing when you're more committed to the problem than to the solution as well as tactics for shifting your energy and attention to implementing effective solutions.

I'm talking from experience here. I caught myself in this uncomfortable, unproductive trap not long ago. The problems I was experiencing were very real, but the solutions were real, too. But I was giving *way* more energy to the problem than to the solution.

Not surprisingly, solutions don't create themselves while we complain about the problem.

In mid-2017, I decided to have a tiny house custom built in Utah and delivered to me in Massachusetts. It was scheduled to arrive just two days before Christmas and I was beyond excited to start a new adventure and a simpler, happier chapter of my life. I invested a lot of time, energy, and money in this new home.

I thought the experience would teach me about simplicity and the important things in life, but it taught me far more than that, largely because of a host of unexpected problems. Without a doubt, it was one of the most challenging experiences of my life.

The problems started before I even took possession of the house. One night, the driver of the truck that was moving my home to Massachusetts called me while I was out to dinner with my boyfriend and his family. The driver was furious. He angrily exclaimed that the builder had given him the wrong dimensions for the house so the transport permits were all wrong, he was breaking the law by even being on the road, and, to make matters worse, he ripped off my home's exterior lights while driving through a toll booth. I was confused, alarmed, and unsure of what to do.

That was only the beginning. I thought I'd be relieved when the house finally got to me, but little did I know we hadn't even scratched the surface of the issues with the home. For months, new problems unfolded every day.

The plumbing was back-pitched and had to be replaced. A large appliance had not been properly secured, so it fell in transit, damaging walls, the floor, and two doorframes.

The media center was built so poorly it had to be torn out. The heating system they installed didn't work when temperatures fell below thirty degrees, which was a bit of a problem since I live in New England. The shower tiles were cracked, the windows didn't fit the window frames, and the hot water didn't run into the kitchen. I documented over four pages of problems, big and small.

I complained about it nonstop, to anyone who would listen. I had decided I was a victim.

Why? Because I wanted to be validated. I felt so wronged and taken advantage of and, to be blunt, the sympathy felt good. Getting people to agree with me about the injustice felt good. I was focused on *being* right instead of *getting* it right. I was angry and I didn't want to be anything else.

Being right required that I prove that the builder and the driver were wrong. Being right wasn't in any way related to actually solving the problems.

In short, I was wasting time, energy, and emotion on something that didn't solve my problems, even though that was all I wanted—solutions! Yes, I wanted solutions, but I wasn't doing anything to create them. The more I shared the problems, the more upset I became. Keeping my attention on the problem made things far worse because it poured gasoline on a fire of negative emotion.

One of the things I teach in my Breaking Barriers e-course is that the lifespan of an emotion is only about ninety seconds. That's right—from the initial burst of anger, sadness, or joy, that emotion has made its full and complete run through your nervous system in ninety seconds or less.

That being true, why do you feel emotions for so much longer than that? Why do you feel angry or frustrated for hours, days, weeks, or even months? Because you keep the emotions alive with your *attention*. In fact, the *only* way to keep them alive is with your attention. Your thoughts and words make them grow.

More importantly, **when your eyes are on the problems, they aren't on the solutions.**

One morning, after discovering a new problem with the house, I told my boyfriend about it. He was mad. He started ranting about what a nightmare this was, how negligent the company was in the construction of the home, and how I had wasted so much time and money.

Like any good hypocrite, I got mad at *him* for responding that way. All I wanted from him were solutions and he had offered none.

I wanted to tell him to either help or shut up, but I couldn't.

I couldn't because I realized that I had been doing the same thing for *months*.

After all, why was he so mad? Because I had been making everyone around me mad about this house. I had riled them all up with my constant complaining.

If I was going to change the situation and get serious about solving problems instead of merely complaining about them, I had to change my attitude.

In order to be part of the solution, I had to stop being part of the problem.

I turned to my boyfriend and calmly said, "I don't want to give any more attention to the problem. I'm only interested in solutions. If you can help me with solutions, awesome. Otherwise, don't allow me to vent about the problem and don't you complain about the problems. Solutions only from here on out."

I started to take the same approach with all my friends and family when they'd call and say, "This is awful! You got screwed!" I calmly replied, "I know I've been complaining nonstop but I'm done with that. I'm not interested in the problem anymore. If you want to help me solve these problems, great. I'm all ears. But if you just want to talk about the problem, I can't join you. I have a finite amount of energy and attention, and I'm only giving it to solutions.

I decided that I wanted solutions more than I wanted attention, and I had to start acting like it.

I called the owner of the manufacturing company and told him the same thing. We were clear on the problems. What could we do that day, right then, to move forward with solutions? What were our options? How could we make this right?

I swallowed my pride and said, "I don't need to be right about what happened and I don't care whose fault it is. I just want to fix it."

I won't tell you that was easy—my ego still wanted to prove that I was right, but I wanted **solutions** more than I wanted to be right, and I knew I had to choose between the two.

When I made that shift, I immediately felt less stressed, more peaceful, and dramatically more in control of the situation.

There was a noticeable change in the builder as well. He became less defensive, less combative, and more willing to participate in fixing the issues. He was proposing solutions instead of defending himself and his company.

Switching to an exclusive focus on the solution made it easier for everyone involved.

You have the ability to do this in *every* situation you're in as well.

You always have a choice: give your energy to the problem or to the solution. You can give your energy to complaining, justifying, and explaining or you can get to work doing something about it.

I can't tell you how many people email me describing the problems in their lives. They're building a case for the problem, justifying it, explaining it, adding layers of detail and substantiation.

They *say* they're looking for help, but you wouldn't know it from their emails. There's no attention, energy, or action going to the solution.

With clients I have history with, I'll often email back and say, "I can't find the part in your email about your role in the solution. Please resend."

It's said with lots of love, but the point is clear—we can't create solutions until we step beyond the problem.

Here's one of the most dangerous parts of giving

your energy to the problems: **you step out of your power.**

When I was focused on everything that was wrong with my house, I had no power. I was simply a victim. I didn't create the problems. They were already done.

In reality, I had a lot of power. I had all the power I needed. I could hire someone to fix the problems. I could sue the builder. I could fix things myself. I could sell the house. Or I could continue to complain about how unfair it all was.

You are powerless in the problem. You are powerful in the solution.

Let's say you work at a job where colleagues are always bringing in fast food and desserts. You work crazy hours and the job is super stressful. There's food everywhere, always, and you feel like you can't overcome the constant temptation.

Got it. The problem is clear. But you don't have a lot of power when you're focused on it.

You step into your power and influence when you focus on the solution. There's so much you *can* control, even in situations where factors are outside of your control. No matter what foods are around you, you're in control of what you put in your mouth, how much, and when. No matter what has been brought in, you don't have to eat it. In fact, it's incredible real-world practice. You wouldn't be able to develop the skills you need for resisting temptation (which is a much needed real-world skill) if you worked in a place *without* such temptations. With that perspective, it's not a problem at all! It's an opportunity!

If you're giving energy to the problem, you're stealing it from the solution.

There will always be things you can't control, and always things you can. Control what you can control. Give your attention to those things.

Break the addiction of talking about problems. Break the habit of complaining. It's making things harder and preventing you from participating in solutions.

If you aren't sure if you're giving attention and energy to the problems, here are some ways it commonly shows up:

- Complaining
- Talking about past failures
- Describing how you struggle
- Explaining the *why* behind the struggle
- Gossiping
- Comparing yourself to other people

- Stressing about future obstacles

It's really **anything that is unrelated to what you are able and willing to do to create a change or improvement.**

I heard about a high school principal who was committed to creating a culture of solution-seeking in his school. When a teacher came to the principal complaining about a student who was rude and disrupting the classroom, the principal was quick to point out that the teacher was merely describing the problem.

The principal took seriously his role in helping the teacher focus on creating solutions. It was clear that the teacher understood the problem, but *reaching* a solution requires participating in it.

The principal asked, "What is your role in this problem? What are possible solutions? What ideas do you have for making a change? What's within your power in terms of creating a change?"

The message was clear: either you're committed to the problem or you're committed to the solution. **Do not come to me to argue for a problem. Come to me to participate in a solution.**

I have similar conversations with my clients every day.

It's not that I don't care to hear about problems, it's that **progress can only come from taking action to participate in a solution.**

When my clients present their problems, I often respond, with a smile, "So what? Now what?"

It's my way of saying, "Okay. I understand. So what will you do about it now?"

The problem isn't limiting your solutions. Your attachment to the problem is what's limiting your solutions.

Remember: transformation is now.

The solution is not a destination; it is a decision. You don't need to wish for it; you need to work for it. Control the controllables.

IN THE STANDS OR IN THE GAME?

I remember a conference leader once quizzing her audience about the difference between a sports spectator and a player in the game. As a group, we brainstormed some of the differences.

Spectators are giving instructions to people in the game. Most of their communication is emotional. They blame and criticize the players—the people doing the work—while they do none. They are talking about what is happening but they aren't doing anything about it. **They can't impact the outcome.**

Players, on the other hand, are *involved*. They're in the moment. They are participating—they're *doing* work instead of talking about it. They are focused on what can be done **now**. There's no focus on yesterday or tomorrow. They're making moves. They have the ability to impact the outcome, and that's where their energy goes.

In your own quest to create change, are you in the stands or are you in the game?

A PROBLEM WELL PUT IS HALF-SOLVED

This isn't just a cute saying; it's also a powerful instruction. A problem well put is half-solved. If you are thinking about or sharing your problems with no mention of what you can do to participate in the solutions, you have work to do.

"I waste too much time on social media" is not a problem well put. It's certainly not half-solved. "I'm going to stay off Facebook tonight" addresses both the problem and the solution.

If you want a solution, don't worry about proving the

severity of the problem and marinating in your feelings about it.

In my own life, I have developed this as a mantra: **I am exclusively focused on solutions.**

When I find myself thinking or talking about how much work I have to do, I remind myself that I am exclusively focused on solutions. Fretting over the workload actually keeps me from creating the solution! What will I do now or next to address the amount of work before me?

I am powerless in the problem. All of my power is in my creation of the solution.

When I find myself thinking or talking about how tired I am, I remind myself that I am exclusively focused on solutions. What am I able and willing to do to increase my energy or prioritize rest?

When I find myself thinking or talking about how stressed I am, I remind myself that I am exclusively focused on solutions. What changes can I make to reduce stress or change my perspective about it?

I am capable of finding, creating, or implementing a solution. What will that take? How can I do it?

You are capable of finding, creating, or implementing a solution. What will that take? How can you do it?

CREATE CHANGE CHALLENGE

Identify a problem, challenge, or area of your life where you desire to create change. For the next three days, be **exclusively** a creative, energetic problem solver. Redirect all thoughts about your problem to action invested in the solution. Choose to have a great attitude, refuse to complain, and take repeated action as often as your time allows. In order to execute this challenge, take a minute to brainstorm distinctions between the problem and the solution.

What is the problem?

How have you been focused on the problem?

How can you participate in the solution?

What options are there?

What factors are unrelated to the solution?

In what situations am I tempted to focus on the problem?

What can I do instead?

Once you're clear on the problem, only allow yourself to be a creative, energetic problem solver! Recruit whatever resources you need to make this happen!

THIRTEEN

Fear of Missing Out

If I say yes to this, what am I saying no to?

One of the most insidious and regret-inducing barriers to change is **fear of missing out**, also known as FOMO. No one describes FOMO better than personal development author Brené Brown, in her book, *Rising Strong*:

> Fear of missing out is what happens when scarcity slams into shame. FOMO lures us out of our integrity with whispers about what we could or should be doing. FOMO's favorite weapon is comparison. It kills gratitude and replaces it with "not enough". We answer FOMO's call by saying YES when we mean NO. We abandon our path and our boundaries and those precious adventures that hold meaning for us so we can prove that we aren't missing out. But we are. We're missing out on our own lives. Every time we say YES because we are afraid of missing out, we say NO to something.

To effectively break down the barrier of FOMO, we must first clarify this idea of "fear." Can we begin by agreeing that fear is *not* the same as danger? Danger represents an immediate and real threat. It's *not* imagined. When a lion is chasing you, you are in danger. Experiencing fear does not mean you are in danger. More often than not, fear actually has nothing to do with danger.

When we aren't thinking clearly, we convince ourselves that we need to respond to fear in the same way we'd respond to danger. We convince ourselves that we need to take immediate action to avoid harm. While that is likely the case with danger, it's not so with fear.

You do not need to act in response to fear. Fear is the *anticipation* of danger or loss. Anticipation is the work of your imagination. **While danger reflects your circumstances, fear reflects your thoughts.** It's all in your head. Fear of missing out is something that comes from your imagination, not from your reality. It is a perception problem.

When you make a choice only to avoid missing out, you're deciding based on an imaginary possibility you invented with your thoughts.

Fortunately, because you are the thinker (you are *not* your thoughts), you can *choose* to change your perception.

FOMO is fueled by a perspective of scarcity. You come into a situation choosing to think that what you have right now isn't enough. You associate loss with not getting more.

You might convince yourself that it isn't enough to enjoy a healthy meal with your friends. You need appetizers, drinks, or dessert to make it better.

It's not enough to window-shop as you explore a new town. You need *more* to make the trip better. You need to buy things.

This way of thinking is not only a lie, it's a vicious cycle. You're not focused on what you *do* have; you're focused only on what you don't have.

Combat FOMO by choosing to think in complete thoughts, rather than incomplete thoughts. What is it that you're afraid to lose? What do you fear missing out on? What will "more" add to your life? Might it actually take something away?

Challenge yourself to tell the truth, even if it hurts, instead of continuing to talk yourself into incomplete truths that feel good for a moment.

Have you ever given in to the idea that indulging would

be better than not indulging, only to wake up the next day regretting all the food you ate?

Have you ever given in to the idea that spending more would make an experience better, only to wake up the next day feeling burdened by the financial pressure you created?

In hindsight, you realize that thing you were so sure would make your experience better actually made it worse.

That's the lie of FOMO.

This was certainly true for my sister Debi and her perspective on spending money. Until she stepped back to question the way she had been thinking, she convinced herself that spending more meant enjoying life more. What was actually true was that spending more was *taking* more from her than it was giving to her. Her lies about money went unexamined for so long that she genuinely believed them. Turns out that spending less removed so much stress and pressure that she was able to enjoy every aspect of her life dramatically more!

Challenge yourself to examine the complete truth. You can choose, by thinking differently, to free yourself from this story of "missing out."

One of the most effective ways to change your perspective is by asking better questions.

If you say yes to this, what are you saying no to?

Use your past experience to debunk the idea of scarcity.

Have you made this choice before?

Was it worth it?

How did you feel the following day?

In your mind, fast-forward twenty-four hours. Which choice would make you feel best: saying yes or saying no?

Are you making a decision based on a fraction of reality?

Are you selling yourself a story simply to justify what you want right now?

What will happen if you continue to make this kind of choice?

If you showed up in this moment as the very best version of yourself, what choice would you make?

These questions continue to be my most-utilized tools

to avoid morning regret. I can't tell you how many times I've woken up the morning after overeating and almost immediately thought, *Why did I do that? It totally wasn't worth it! It's never worth it!*

I shudder to think how many times I woke up wishing I could undo the previous night's food choices and beating myself up for going overboard again.

I hate that feeling.

So, when evening fatigue starts to impair my decision-making and I'm considering turning to food when I don't need it, I think ahead to the next morning. If I make this choice, how will I feel about it tomorrow? Do I want to feel that way? Is it worth it? What would it take for me to wake up feeling amazing? Do I want that?

Will I act like it?

Think back to Brené Brown's description of FOMO. "We abandon our path and our boundaries and those precious adventures that hold meaning for us so we can prove that we aren't missing out. But we are. We're missing out on our own lives."

If you continue to say yes to that temptation, what will you miss?

Is it worth it?

Is there something that means more to you than this temptation?

Is your dream for sale?

Are you acting like it?

Fear of missing out was a big part of why I gave myself permission to go overboard on vacations, business trips, or even just weekends and evenings out! I'd tell myself I wanted to relax, let loose, and treat myself.

I convinced myself that a low-key weekend wasn't enough—I needed more. I convinced myself that I could increase the pleasurability of the experience by over-indulging. The pleasure was always disappointingly short-lived.

Overeating wasn't relaxing. It created endless stress. I wasn't treating myself. I was keeping myself in a prison I was desperate to escape.

Saying yes to overeating meant saying no to feeling great. Saying yes to all the food meant saying no to making progress toward the weight loss goal that meant so much to me. Saying yes to overindulging meant saying no to feeling amazing the next day.

Saying yes to indulgence meant chasing pleasure at the expense of happiness.

I was abandoning the path that held so much meaning—getting healthy and creating confidence—just so I could avoid missing out on more food. Meanwhile, I was missing out on the life that was possible for me.

At some point, I had to acknowledge that there really wasn't anything special about another basket of tortilla chips, bowl of ice cream, or plate of pancakes. These things had nothing more to offer me. I wasn't going to continue to tell myself that the couple minutes of pleasure were worth missing out on the life I wanted.

Once I acknowledged the trade I had been making, I could see through the lie of FOMO. It no longer had a hold on me. Brutal honesty removed the appeal of all those things that captivated me for decades.

Train your brain, by asking better questions, to see all sides of the FOMO thought process, not just that well-worn permissive path. That is the essence of your work here as you break these barriers to change. You're becoming a better, more honest, and complete thinker.

YOLO, AN EVIL TWIN OF FOMO

Not long ago, I was on a short ski vacation in Maine. My boyfriend and I went up for a weekend and his father joined us for one night.

The three of us went out to dinner and I happily ordered a large salad and glass of water. When we finished our meals, the waitress asked if we'd like any dessert. My boyfriend's father asked for the brownie sundae with three spoons—one for each of us. "None for me," I said. "I'm all set."

With a knowing smile he said, "Oh no, you're going to have some! We're on vacation. You only live once!"

YOLO. You only live once. You've probably heard that before.

It's absolutely true, to my knowledge, that I only live once. I spent most of my life using FOMO and YOLO to justify overindulging. To justify anything I wanted, really. It was an *awful* strategy. It didn't work for me. It didn't make me happy. It didn't get me what I want in life. In fact, it kept me *from* it! Using that line to talk myself into overeating brought me to a place where I was hardly living at all. I was very much alive but very much *not* living.

Here's what I have decided is true for me: *since* I only live once, I don't want to miss out on confidence. I don't want to miss out on feeling great in my body. I don't want to miss out on energy and vitality. I don't want to miss out on adventures.

I am happy to "miss out" on binging, overeating, drinking too much, and tasting every treat that is offered to me.

Redefine what *you* don't want to miss. Since you only live once, how do you want to live?

What drives your choices? Are you focused on what you want *most* or what you want *now*?

A few bites of a brownie sundae wasn't going to add anything to my life or my vacation, but an operating system of always saying yes to indulging and no to my goals would certainly *take* something from my life.

When you say yes to one thing, you're saying no to something else.

The brownie sundae came and I didn't eat it. I didn't feel like I was missing out because of the perspective I chose. In fact, I've used the power of my thoughts (combined with an honest evaluation of my past experiences) to convince myself that I'd actually miss out more if I chose to have the sundae.

Practice seeking the *complete* version of your truth.

WHOLE AND UNDIVIDED

One of the concepts that has been instrumental in helping me develop immunity to FOMO is something I found in a definition of the word "integrity."

I've often defined integrity as a habit of keeping the promises you make and holding true to your word even when no one is watching. From that perspective, integrity sounds a lot like discipline, which is undoubtedly accurate. However, lately I've been more drawn to this definition:

Integrity is the state of being whole and undivided.

The feeling of FOMO waves a warning flag that you aren't thinking in a whole and undivided way.

You have one foot in your past and one in your future. You can't live your best life when you're divided.

For most of my life I was anything *but* whole and undivided. I wanted to be healthy and happy, yet I was choosing things that didn't make me healthy or happy. There was a wide gap between who I was and who I wanted to be. There were miles between my intentions and my actions. I was dramatically divided and felt broken on every level.

Overeating because I didn't want to miss out came with a tremendous amount of tension—I felt torn between my goals and my desires. If one won, I felt the other had to lose.

The view of integrity as being whole and undivided gave me a lot to think about.

What does it mean to me? I want to be someone who can indulge without guilt and also without excess. I want to be someone who feels amazing about all my choices.

I want to be someone who can pour myself fully into my work and also make time for friends, family, and fun.

When I feel little twinges of FOMO, I ask myself what choice I could make that would leave me feeling whole and undivided.

I began asking myself what it could look like **to live peacefully with all that I desire.** No FOMO. No guilt.

I don't have to live in deprivation and I also don't have to submit to gluttony. I don't have to fear missing out because there is a way to live peacefully with all I desire.

Let's be honest—I wasn't 350 pounds because every once in a while I enjoyed a decadent indulgence. I was

350 pounds because I indulged too often, I took it too far, and I regularly ate things that weren't worth it.

People routinely ask me how I handle feeling guilty when I drink alcohol or eat cupcakes. The honest answer is that I don't feel guilty at all. I am not striving to be a perfectionist. I am not striving to be someone who never indulges. I am striving to be someone who indulges in a way that still makes me feel amazing and honors my goals. I indulge when it's worth it and I avoid taking it to the extent or frequency that it makes me feel bad. When it's not worth it, I don't indulge.

Remember that binary can be the opposite of creativity. You don't have to decide between loving your work and loving your family. You don't have to decide between financial freedom and your dream vacation. You don't have to decide between sugar and health.

Take a few minutes to think about the area (or areas) in which you want to make progress. Whether it's your weight, health, self-talk, fitness, career, finances, or relationships, what does it look like for you to feel and be whole and undivided? If you went through an entire day (or week) in a way that felt whole and undivided, what would it look like? Be as specific as possible.

Perhaps more importantly, what does it look like for you

to *not* be whole and undivided? Where do you show up, choose, or behave in a way that doesn't reflect the person you want to be? What does it look like when you're not acting with integrity?

CREATE CHANGE CHALLENGE

Reverse your perspective on missing out. Set a timer for five minutes and sit without interruption. Consider your answers to the following question:

In what areas of your life do you most frequently say yes when you mean no? Be as specific as possible.

For example, "When I say yes to overeating on the weekend, I say no to feeling great, I say no to starting the week well, and I say no to my weight loss goal."

Or "When I say yes to being condescending or dismissive to my partner, I say no to having a great night with him/her. I say no to getting closer and really connecting."

Once you have identified one or two scenarios where you are too often saying yes instead of no, go through the questions in this chapter to see the situation in a more honest light. Reframe the idea of missing out.

- What do you want most?

- Why do you want it?
- What's the downside to saying yes to those things?
- What's the upside to saying no?
- When will you practice saying no instead of yes?
- How will you recognize the lie of FOMO the next time it comes up?

FOURTEEN

Change Your Reputation

"Self-esteem is just the reputation that you have with yourself."

—NAVAL RAVIKANT

When you repeatedly let yourself down, you sacrifice your self-esteem. Self-esteem, as Ravikant explains, is the reputation you have with yourself. The disappointment, frustration, and doubt that come from repeated excuses and exceptions begin to shape the way you see yourself. More appropriately, they begin to limit the way you see yourself.

One of the most common things I observe in emails from clients who are struggling is that they have begun to define themselves based on what they *don't* want. Whether they feel they're an all-or-nothing person, describe themselves as inconsistent, or state that they're an emotional eater, the pattern is clear: they identify with a reputation of themselves that has tremendous room for improvement.

Fortunately, who you think you are is not a fixed position. You can change it, and it's much easier than you might think.

There are thousands of books on the market that appeal to readers because they attempt to help them understand themselves and their choices. To do that, these books assign personality types. They place people in predefined categories. These books say to the reader, "You behave this way because you are this type of person. You continue to struggle with this thing because you are that type of person." We breathe a sigh of relief. It's not that we are weak or unmotivated...it's just who we are. It's our personality.

To varying extents, we use these personality types to let ourselves off the hook and justify our patterns. The dangerous trap, however, is that it can take us out of our power and prevent us from taking the responsibility required to create meaningful change. We begin to believe in these artificial constraints.

Within the framework of whatever personality type you

think you are, you now have something on which to pin your habits. "It's because I'm a rebel!"

Let's shoot straight, shall we? **You are whatever you decide to be.** The only limits on your behavior come from your own choices. Who you were yesterday or that pattern of behavior you think defines you—it's all changeable.

An introvert can choose to be something else, if they so desire.

A motivated person can choose to be lazy.

A liar can choose to be honest.

A quitter can see something through.

A genius can get it all wrong.

You can be a rule follower *and* a rule breaker. You can be externally *and* internally motivated. You choose! You don't just choose once. You choose every day, in every moment that you make a choice.

Your behavioral tendencies are not who you are—and you can change them. Your habits aren't your only options. Your past is a memory; it is not a projection.

There is no behavioral pattern that can't be changed.

In any and every moment, you have the opportunity to change your own reputation.

When change feels hard and you're overwhelmed by the idea of it, here's what can set you free:

You are the solution you've been waiting for. You are only one choice away from creating a new pattern or establishing a new reputation.

Just because you've always been an emotional eater doesn't mean you can't be something else.

Just because you've always been a workaholic doesn't mean you can't change that reputation and create a new reality. Every day is a chance to do just that.

Think about someone you know who has a bad reputation. How did they get that reputation? Their choices, right? Reputation stems from one's repeated actions.

Can they change it? Yes!

Your reputation reflects your patterns of behavior and the extent to which there is congruence between what you say and what you do. **While your reputation is**

influenced by your past, it's not limited by it. If your reputation doesn't reflect who or how you want to be, you can go about changing it the same way anyone else would.

What would it take for a person with a lousy reputation to change it? How could they go about repairing their relationship with you and restoring trust? What would they have to do to change the way you see them?

They would have to consistently choose improved behaviors and also avoid the negative behaviors that led to the poor reputation in the first place. They'd have to show initiative. Once or twice wouldn't be enough. It wouldn't be sufficient for them to act differently only when they feel like it.

How would you feel if someone close to you pledged to improve their reputation and change their behavior but kept putting it off?

If it's not acceptable for them, why would you accept it from yourself?

Keep these things in mind as you now think about your own reputation. I don't want you to think about how others see you—**exclusively consider how you see yourself.**

As it relates to the primary goal you are pursuing or the

change you're trying to create, what is the reputation you have with yourself now? In what ways would you like to change it?

Take a few minutes to answer as specifically as possible.

- Is your reputation that you're lazy and inconsistent?
- Do you lack follow-through?
- Do you make a lot of excuses?
- What are the excuses you make?
- Do you cut corners? In what ways?
- What would you like your reputation to be?
- How do you want to see yourself?
- How do you want others to see you?
- Are you willing to do the work and be the change?

I'm going to give you a tool you can use every time you're frustrated with yourself or feel tempted to submit to habits you're trying to break. If you commit to practicing with this tool, you'll be able to cut through the emotional entanglement of past patterns in record time. You'll slash through the drama and delay in your life. This is the tool you'll use to close the gap between the reputation you presently have and the one you want to create. As you bridge the gap, your self-esteem will improve and your choices will improve right along with it!

The tool comes in the form of a question.

What is the behavior you wish you would effortlessly demonstrate in this situation?

If you were the ideal version of yourself—exactly the person you wish to be—what would you do? How would you behave? What choice would you make?

Identify it. Then do it.

My past patterns created an awful reputation with regards to food. I believed that every slip became a slide. I'd intend to eat *so* healthy, but then after eating a donut at work, I'd say, "Screw it! I blew it!" and get candy on the way home from work, order takeout for dinner, and follow it up with a pint of ice cream.

As soon as I indulged during the workday, I'd start to feel myself panic. I was smack in the middle of the emotions I had learned to associate with that pattern of behavior. I didn't want to go down that slippery slope, but it was such a well-worn path I didn't know how to stop myself, either.

Equipped with a deep breath and a blank piece of paper, I'd ask myself that single question.

What is the behavior you wish you'd effortlessly demonstrate in this situation?

I want to be the kind of person who can have a donut in the middle of the day and then go about eating well. No drama. No reason to justify overeating later. No guilt. Just a donut followed by a day of great choices.

Boom. There it is. With that question, I'm never stuck. I can never say that I don't know where to start or how to change. The answer to that question is my compass. It gives me my solution. It lights the path to my new reputation.

I want to be someone who doesn't choose to derail after enjoying a treat.

I wouldn't freak out over whether or not I could behave that way forever. Forever isn't here today. But, just for today, I could be that person—I could show up as that version of myself for a handful of choices.

This was one of the most powerful strategies I used while writing this book. Going into the writing process, the reputation I had with myself was that I have an incredibly short attention span—a lot like that of a fruit fly. I'm easily distracted. I'm either on (writing feels easy) or I'm off (writing is impossible).

When I choose to believe that story, I feel overwhelmed and incapable. The emotions that come along with choosing to think that way impede any and all progress.

Instead of settling into those feelings and believing in my past patterns, I'd snap myself out of the emotions by asking myself, "What is the behavior I wish I would effortlessly demonstrate when I sit down to write?" Or I'd ask, "What kind of writer do I really want to be?"

I want to approach my writing time enthusiastically. I want to be eager to share my thoughts on paper. I want to grab hold of ideas that get me excited and write from the heart. I want to be disciplined and resistant to distractions. I want to be patient with myself while also upholding the kind of work ethic that makes me proud.

Then I'd say to myself, "Great! Practice showing up that way for the next fifteen minutes."

Some days, I'd challenge myself to practice that way of being—creating that new reputation—for twenty or thirty minutes. Other days, I'd start with just five.

Have you heard the cliché "What follows 'I am' follows you?" It's true.

When I tell myself that I'm easily distracted, I give in to distractions.

When I tell myself I am capable of focusing for five minutes, I focus for five minutes.

When I would tell myself that I am an emotional eater, I'd turn to food when I was sad.

When I tell myself that I am capable of taking great care of myself when I'm upset, I do.

That strategy is available to you every day. You can practice when you're aggravated with a coworker or when you're putting off your household chores. You can practice when you're upset with a loved one or when you're facing temptation.

I'm going to guess that some of you are feeling a little skeptical of this strategy. When you're *not* in one of those hard moments, this seems pretty straightforward. But, when in the heart of the struggle, how do you make yourself care enough to practice?

Your skepticism points right at what makes this change feel so hard: emotion.

It's not your past pattern that is the problem. It's not even the reputation you have with yourself as a result of those patterns. It's your feelings about it.

When you strip away the emotion, it's really quite simple.

There's a pattern of behavior that isn't working for you.

You wish you were the type of person who _____.

However you fill in that sentence is exactly the thing you need to do.

Simple!

But you cannot *see* the simplicity when your attention and energy are being poured into how you *feel* about the problem.

You can't identify and act upon the simple solution when you're in your feelings. That's why this is a practice.

Don't forget what we talked about in Part One. Customer service is an inside job. The solution is right here at your fingertips; you have to move out of the sensing stage and right into the solving stage. Commit to recognizing when you're marinating in your feelings about the problem. That's not where the solution is.

The solution is right over here, out of the muck of your emotions, right in this simple space.

Identify who and how you want to be. Then act that way.

You aren't pledging a permanent change. You're choosing a single response.

This is your practice. The more you embrace it, the more quickly it will become a pattern. As it becomes a pattern, your own reputation will shift and improve. Your confidence will grow.

One of my Primal Potential Masters Club clients recently updated our Facebook group with how things are going for her...kind of. She told us that most of her time and energy is going into thinking but not doing. She described a significant mismatch between her actions and her intentions.

Her comments didn't include anything about the solution or the action she could take. She was merely sharing, and therefore reinforcing, the problem.

I brought this to her attention. She was building a case for that reputation she doesn't want—she's a thinker, not a doer. I challenged her, as I do most of my clients.

"You are free to change this reputation. Instead of bemoaning the existing reputation, get busy building the new one. What do you want it to be? Fill in this sentence: I wish I were the type of person who _____. Now, your task is to act on what is in that space. Those are your marching orders. Get busy!"

When you find yourself struggling to change, take a step

back and ask yourself if the solution is anywhere in your thoughts or actions. More often than not, it isn't.

What is the behavior you wish you would effortlessly demonstrate in this situation?

That's your work. That's how you'll close the gap between the way you've been and the way you wish to be.

CREATE CHANGE CHALLENGE

It's time to change the reputation you have with yourself.

- Who do you want to be?
- How do you want to be?
- How does the person you want to be act?
- What choices do they make?
- What choices do they not make?

Sit with your journal and write out what it will take for you to change your reputation. Be as specific as possible. Every day for one week, begin your morning by identifying the specific steps you'll take that day to create your improved reputation.

Every time you are caught up in the appeal of a past pattern, pause to ask and answer, "What is the behavior I wish I would effortlessly demonstrate in this situation?"

After each day has wrapped, review it. How did you feel? What worked? What didn't? How could you have made it better? What will you incorporate tomorrow? What did you learn?

Every morning, revisit the ideas of who and how you want to be. Continue to reinforce in your thoughts and actions the type of person you desire to be.

FIFTEEN

Navigate the Darkness

"If you lose the spirit of repetition your practice will become quite difficult."

—SHUNRYU SUZUKI

If your goal is to create lasting change in your life, you must *use* the dark and difficult moments to practice consistency. Don't resent these moments. **They are not here to give you an excuse to run from progress.** The hard moments are an essential part of your process. Hard moments, hard days, and even hard years are part of the human experience. You can't avoid them.

You can decide to abandon your goals and self-care during these times, you can continue to let your circumstances determine your choices, *or* you can practice being someone who remains in control of your choices regardless of your external circumstances.

You can merely survive the dark moments, you can submit to them and let them run your life, or you can choose to thrive in the midst of them.

Will you be someone who does what is right or someone who does what is easy? Will you be someone who makes yourself a victim of your circumstances or you will you choose to be victorious despite them?

It's easy to convince yourself that there isn't time or energy for your goals when you're going through something challenging. You can convince yourself that you simply *can't* take great care of yourself when life is hard. But you can.

I have a lot of experience letting emotion, loss, fatigue, and stress be the reasons I didn't take care of myself. I convinced myself that it was too hard. The **real** truth is that *not* taking care of myself made the hard times harder. On the flip side, maintaining consistency and making great choices no matter what is happening in my life makes the hard times easier. There have been no exceptions to this rule.

These days, when I'm super stressed or life feels out of

control, I remind myself: **this is when it matters most.** This is when my choices need to be the very best, not the very worst!

While this might sound reasonable in theory, what you choose in practice is what matters most. You have to take this from idea to execution. How can you convince yourself to endure those moments when you simply want to quit and can make a solid case for easing off or giving up?

Some of the most helpful advice I've ever heard on this topic came from Olympic gymnast Nastia Liukin.

Nastia's gymnastics career began when she was just three years old. By the time she was in grade school, she was already a full-time athlete. As if that's not challenging enough, her own father was her coach. The demands of her training were often overwhelming. Many days, she'd cry to her mother that she wanted to quit. She didn't want to be a gymnast anymore.

Her mother's response was both brilliant and instructive. "You can absolutely quit," she'd say. "You don't have to do this. But, you can't quit on a bad day. Wait until you have a good day; then you can quit."

Inevitably, Nastia would come home energized and

excited after nailing a new skill or having a great training day and her mom would ask, "So, do you still want to quit?"

On a good day, the answer was always no.

In your own life, **never quit on a bad day.** Never give up because you're frustrated, tired, or stressed. Never give up because you aren't seeing progress. Never.

Remember the Jocko Willink advice we talked about? Emotion doesn't get a vote. Frustration doesn't get a vote. Temptation doesn't get a vote.

Having struggled with my weight for my entire life, I was a chronic quitter. One of the primary reasons change felt so hard was that I always entertained quitting as an option. I had a well-worn pattern of giving up as soon as things got hard. For most of my life, no diet survived a terrible day or emotional overload. Unlike Nastia, I quit when it felt too hard.

I used food to self-medicate and distract myself from every negative emotion. Every hard moment and unexpected event was a reason to throw in the towel on personal responsibility and self-discipline. I convinced myself that I was too emotional to make a great choice or that overeating would make me feel better.

But feeling *less* isn't the same as feeling *better*.

It didn't work. It was the easy choice and my most familiar, practiced response.

I wasn't solving problems by turning to food; I was creating new ones. Overeating in response to stress or sadness meant that I was not only sad or stressed, but also disappointed and disgusted with myself.

Thanks to Liukin's mother's approach, I now see it differently. I can absolutely quit, and so can you, but only on a good day.

Refuse to give in or give up on a bad day. Remind yourself that on those bad days, your emotional filter is clouding your vision. Wait it out and hang in there until you have a good day.

Better yet, *create* a great day and revisit the decision then.

Don't deviate from your commitments on a bad day. Don't let a bad moment erase your good intentions. That's the rule.

A few weeks ago, I was craving pancakes. I can't tell you the last time I had pancakes, but for some reason, they suddenly sounded like the very best food on the planet.

After a few days of continuously thinking about how delicious they would be, I decided that I would in fact enjoy a big plate of pancakes the following Saturday. But, I told myself, in the meantime, I had to create great days. Yes, I could savor those pancakes the following weekend, but between now and then, I had to make all my food choices winning choices that made me feel proud.

Throughout the week, I built momentum. I made great choice after great choice and I was feeling *really* good! Saturday morning came and I went to the gym first thing. As I was leaving, having had a great workout and a solid week of awesome choices, I thought, *I don't even want those pancakes! It feels so great to feel this good; the pancakes just aren't worth it!*

It wasn't that I no longer desired pancakes, I just wanted to feel incredible *more* than I wanted to taste pancakes.

Create some space between yourself and your urge to indulge or give up. You aren't telling yourself no, you're just making sure you decide from a brighter state of mind. Use your great choices to make yourself feel better (even if you're already feeling good). Then, make the decision when you feel amazing.

One of my clients shared with me that she and her husband have a household rule: **they don't drink alcohol when they are sad.**

They do drink, and love to enjoy cocktails together, but it's not something they will turn to in a negative emotional state. They don't drink after a bad day at work, a financial setback, or a loss in their family.

I started practicing a similar rule a couple years ago: **I don't indulge alone.** If I'm going to indulge in alcohol or food, I just don't do it alone. I won't eat in my car; I won't eat a pint of ice cream alone on the couch. I won't stock up on cookies and chips at the grocery store and binge by myself while watching Netflix.

As someone who used to sneak food and overindulge when no one was looking, this has been a huge area of growth for me. *Pleasure shared is pleasure multiplied.* If I want something, I refuse to hide it.

These are all variations of that powerful idea: refuse to quit on a bad day.

I'm not suggesting either of those are the right approaches for you, but I do think **not quitting on a bad day** is one we can all grow from.

I want to help you shift your perspective about the hard

moments you *will* face so they don't continue to fuel excuses and inconsistency.

It's often most tempting to overeat, overspend, or drink too much when life feels hard. However, those behaviors aren't solutions; they are distractions.

More often than not, they not only fail to make the situation better, they actually make it *worse*.

Instead of just being stressed or overwhelmed, you create a situation where the negativity is now compounded with frustration, fatigue, disappointment, shame, and lethargy. In addition to feeling bad about your circumstances, you now also feel bad about your choices. Maybe you even feel badly about yourself!

At the highest level, you always have the power to make the hard times worse or make them better.

Turning away from self-care makes it worse. Making excuses and throwing in the towel erodes your energy and confidence. It darkens your mood.

One of the darkest times in my life was when I separated from my husband. I had recently quit my job to launch Primal Potential. The company wasn't yet making money. I had no income, no health insurance, was living fifteen hours away from my family while trying to navigate a heartbreaking transition.

There were many moments when I told myself I didn't have the emotional bandwidth to prioritize things like nutrition and exercise. I wanted to throw in the towel and distract myself with ice cream and pizza. I doubt anyone would have blamed me.

Here's the critical piece of reality that thinking in complete thoughts reminded me: letting myself go, even for a day, would have made a hard situation worse.

It would have compounded my struggle and made every day *more* difficult. It would have added frustration, disappointment, and fear to my sadness, grief, and confusion.

Avoiding self-care isn't a survival mechanism—it's destruction. It is dangerously shortsighted.

On the flip side, my decision to keep nutrition and exercise at the top of my priority list made that dark season of life more bearable.

Despite going through emotional and financial turmoil, I felt proud of myself. I trusted myself. I had plenty of energy. I was encouraged by my progress and that kept me going. I was building my confidence instead of eroding it.

I had a choice and so do you. You can return to past patterns, distract yourself, and play the victim card. It won't make life easier; it will make it harder.

You're not giving yourself a break; you're breaking yourself down.

Alternatively, you can be militantly on your own side.

You can see your challenging life circumstances as reasons why you can't take care of yourself or you can see them as reasons why you must.

In that dark season of life, each time I considered turning to food or alcohol, I told myself to **hold steady**. Keep making the right choice, one choice at a time, until the tide turns. Don't stop. Never quit on a bad day.

I chose to make myself better instead of resigning to making myself feel worse. I refused to betray myself.

Life will be hard, my friend. There will be high highs and there will be low lows. The times when you don't think you can take great care of yourself are the times when it matters most that you do.

As I was making the final edits to this book, I took a break to watch a Patriots football game. The Pats were down in the second half when the commentator remarked that no team in the NFL has the **competitive stamina** that the Patriots do. They are known to fight until the very last second, no matter how much they are down. That's one of the primary reasons they've had such great success as a franchise. They made the greatest comeback in Super Bowl history, coming back from a 28-3 deficit to beat the Atlanta Falcons 34-28. They refuse to stop fighting, no matter what the scoreboard says.

I'm sure you've seen a sporting event where the losing team stops fighting before the clock expires. They figure that losing is a foregone conclusion and they stop fighting. They lack competitive stamina.

I think we have a tendency to do this in our own lives and it makes change infinitely harder than it needs to be. An unexpected expense comes up so we stop trying to make our budget work for the month. Work stress adds up so we ditch our pledge to work out three days a week. The scale doesn't reflect our hard work so we stop trying to eat healthy and decide to pound a pint of ice cream.

You need to build competitive stamina. The dark and difficult moments are a great chance to do just that. Don't stop fighting. The game is not over; you haven't lost. The only way you'll lose is if you stop fighting.

You can make a comeback. Every choice is a chance.

KNOW WHAT TO IGNORE

I once heard a math teacher explain how he encourages his students to get better at math. He introduces them to a concept he calls "butt power." Yes, you did in fact read that right. Butt power.

You know when you're sitting at your computer facing a problem you can't seem to solve and your instinct is to check Facebook, get a drink of water, go to the bathroom, or start something new?

Enter: butt power. The power to stay right there, on your butt, resisting distractions and continuing to do the work until you break through.

Don't turn away. Don't open Facebook. Don't check your email. Build your butt power.

While that can be super helpful when you're trying to get things done at work, it also applies when you want to turn to food, alcohol, social media, gossip, or spending money to soothe yourself.

Don't.

This is your chance to build your butt power. Sit with the feeling. Don't run from the discomfort.

We often turn to distractions as soon as things start to feel uncomfortable. Sometimes the discomfort comes from temptation, sometimes it comes from fatigue, hunger, loneliness, or frustration.

Instead of riding the wave of the emotion and getting to the other side, we feel compelled to turn away, to react immediately and run from the hard moment.

Don't.

Here's your chance to practice. You have an opportunity to build your butt power. Find out what it feels like to get to the other side *without* running away. Give yourself the experience of watching it fade and subside. Prove to yourself that you can endure that moment without the aid of food, alcohol, or any other distraction.

I practice butt power every chance I get (and I get a lot of chances).

If I'm feeling a little hungry, I'll challenge myself to build butt power. Don't get up and prowl through the fridge,

Elizabeth. Sit with it. You don't need to immediately react. Ride it out.

When I feel mentally stuck when writing and I'm tempted to check email or turn on the news, I challenge myself to build butt power in that moment. Don't click off this page. Ride this out. Stay with the work. This is a chance to practice.

When I'm lonely or tired and I am looking to food for a distraction, I know it's an opportunity to build that butt power. It's a chance to prove to myself that nothing bad will happen if I feel this feeling. I don't have to run from it. I don't have to seek distraction. I'm okay.

If my boyfriend has said something that ruffles my feathers and I want to be rude or snarky, I remind myself that this is a wonderful chance to just sit with it, resist the urge, and build butt power. Stay right here. There's no need to react or distract. This is a chance.

One of the greatest insights you can develop is knowing what to ignore. Is it the urge to snack that you need to ignore? The temptation to gossip? Social media?

What do you need to ignore?

CREATE CHANGE CHALLENGE

The next time you find yourself negotiating for an excuse, exception, or choice that doesn't reflect progress toward your goal, put that decision on hold. Create one amazing day—a day where you feel maximally proud of your choices and decisions.

- What does your amazing day look like?
- When will you execute it, without excuse?
- At the end of your amazing day, when you're feeling proud and encouraged, revisit that choice you were considering.
- Is it still the right one for you?
- How will you feel afterwards?
- Is it worth it?
- What did you learn?

SIXTEEN

Experience Maximum Effort

"Unlearn the habit of living incompletely."

—DANIELLE LAPORTE

Don't mistake the familiarity of your comfort zone with "easy." Don't convince yourself that *not* trying is easier than trying. *Living with an unrealized goal isn't easy at all.* Though living with a struggle might be familiar, it's not your best life. There is so much more available for you and it's time for you to choose it.

Katrin Daviðsdóttir, CrossFit superstar and two-time Fittest Woman on Earth, talks candidly about her life as a professional athlete. She trains intensely for hours every day. She plans her meals and adheres to a very strict diet. She's militant about getting enough sleep. Performing at her level demands that she take impeccable care of her body in a way that requires a tremendous amount of sacrifice. Every aspect of her life revolves around her sport.

Despite the countless sacrifices, I believe her when she says that her very best and happiest days are the ones when she is training hardest and eating cleanest. Nothing is more satisfying and exciting than when she's aggressively pursuing her goals and pushing her limits. Nothing feels better than making progress. She doesn't live for her rest days or light training days. She isn't pining for a cheat meal. She feels her *best* when she is working her hardest.

To be perfectly honest, I think that's true for all of us; we just don't yet know it because we haven't given ourselves that experience. We haven't created an uninterrupted string of days or weeks where we do our best and take impeccable care of ourselves without exception. We don't know how amazing we would feel if we brought our best effort (consistently) and stopped making excuses.

The thrill and pride of progress feels significantly better than the pleasure of indulgence and the familiarity of excuses.

Does this idea remind you of the phrase "nothing tastes as good as thin feels"? As I shared earlier, I hate that phrase and I always have. My mom and grandmother used to say it to me when I was a fat kid who had never been thin. I couldn't even relate. I didn't know what it felt like to be thin, but I knew I certainly loved cupcakes!

However, therein lies my point.

You don't *know* how amazing you can feel and I want you to give yourself that experience. Only then can you make a decision about your best approach. Only then can you have an honest perspective about the appeal of indulgences and "days off."

You can always go back to the way things were. You can return to average. You can go back to kind of trying and living in the middle. You can always go back to making excuses and putting it off, but I need you to at least give yourself the experience of maximum effort so you see how amazing you can feel.

The excitement that comes from watching your body change and the sustained energy that comes from making great choices feels dramatically better than the short-lived pleasure of indulging.

The pride and peace associated with paying off your debt are dramatically more rewarding than the temporary high you get from buying something new.

The confidence that comes from being proud of yourself is immeasurably more satisfying than the short-term relief of procrastination.

What is waiting for you on the other side of the work you're avoiding will feel better than the comfort of where you are right now.

It's okay if you aren't sure about that or haven't ever experienced it. That's precisely the point. Create the experience because you deserve to find out.

Too often, we're either not trying, which sucks, or we're straddling the middle and kind of trying, which also sucks.

There is another option, which is to show up and do your best every single day. Maximum effort.

Work hard and don't take your foot off the gas. Create the change you crave and see how amazing you can feel. See what kind of change you can generate in your life when you actually put your consistent action *and* unwavering effort into it.

Learn what it feels like to do your best, consistently.

I promise you that as you step into the cycle of accelerated returns where you are doing the work, feeling proud, and making progress, you will understand why I'm encouraging it so strongly. It feels amazing.

I remind myself of this often. Every time I'm facing a temptation or considering an excuse, I have an opportunity to practice. Sure, I can convince myself that I just want to have a cupcake or a margarita, but what I know is true is that **my happiest, most pleasant days are when I'm taking impeccable care of my body, my relationships, my work, and my finances.**

I spent most of my life overindulging, making excuses, and living with excess. That was not a happy way of life. In fact, it was miserable.

When I wasn't overeating and overindulging, I was kind of trying. I'd have some good days and some bad days. That didn't feel great either, because I wasn't seeing results.

I still find myself thinking about how amazing it would be to order a pizza, drink margaritas, and zone out with Netflix. I have moments when I daydream about a creamy scoop of ice cream on top of a warm chocolate chip cookie.

Then, I remind myself of the dangers of incomplete thinking. Yes, those things would taste good, but they wouldn't make me *feel* good. They certainly wouldn't make me feel my best, and I want to feel incredible! I am *capable* of making myself feel incredible.

Consistently doing my best gave me the gift of a different version of the truth. A more complete version of the truth—a version that moves me forward. Yes, indulging feels good. *Not* indulging feels so much better!

You're not alone if you think a shopping spree or "cheat day" would be amazing.

It's nowhere *near* as amazing as the excitement you feel when you're impressing yourself, creating change, exceeding your expectations, and improving your life. Momentary indulgences can't hold a candle to building your confidence, stepping into your highest potential, and watching it unfold in front of you. *Making* it unfold.

There is a priceless level of energy and enthusiasm that level of effort brings into your life. I want you to feel it.

It might be helpful to think about this concept in terms of fasting. The first couple days of a water fast are undeniably the hardest. I'd go so far as to say they suck. Most people find that they are uncomfortably hungry and irritable. Not willing to endure the discomfort, they break the fast. Their perspective on fasting is therefore seriously flawed because they only did the hard part. They gave up before it got easier. There's nothing wrong with them for breaking the fast, but the sense that it's "so hard" isn't about the fast—it's about how *they* fasted.

They didn't give themselves the experience of how great it feels once you get *through* the hard part. Hunger subsides, energy soars, and you can feel unstoppable. But most people don't know or believe that because they've never tried it.

The same is true with the experience of maximum effort. Most people don't know how amazing it feels because they don't stick it out long enough to find out.

Be different. Don't quit. You can do it. It is worth it.

This idea might make some of you uncomfortable. It might feel extreme or like the "all" side of all-or-nothing. This actually came up not long ago on one of my client webinars when someone asked what I thought of the concept known as minimum effective dose.

In short, minimum effective dose is the *smallest amount of effort* that will produce your desired result.

My client wanted to know when this minimum effective dose makes sense and when maximum effort is more appropriate.

Here's my take:

You already know what it's like to do the minimum. And maybe you've experienced giving your full, unreserved effort for a few days here and there. But have you ever experienced being consistent in the pursuit of your very best for several uninterrupted weeks? Months? Have you ever done your best and brought your maximum effort *without exception* for an extended period of time?

That's the experience I want you to create for yourself.

It doesn't mean you are forever a perfectionist. It doesn't mean you decide to be a lifelong purist. You don't have to do it until the end of time. I simply want you to see what it feels like to show up, consistently, as the best version of yourself. I want you to create the experience, over a period of *weeks*, where you do your best and entertain no other option.

I want you to see what it feels like to take this approach without complaining and convincing yourself that you're a victim of your own discipline. You're intentionally bringing your best effort because you're worth it and because you want to feel unstoppable. It's the furthest thing from a sacrifice. It's one of the very best gifts you can give yourself.

Then you can answer that minimum effective dose question with a response that is specific to you and not a gross overgeneralization.

Which approach makes *you* feel better? Which approach makes you happiest?

Half-assing it? Doing the minimum amount that sometimes gets some results? Kind of trying? Straddling the middle? Being on again, off again? Or doing your best?

You can always go back to the way things were. You can always stop trying. But living a life where you don't know what it looks or feels like to consistently bring your maximum effort...you're ripping yourself off.

You won't know how bad you feel until you start making yourself feel better. You won't know how much better you can feel until you stop making yourself feel bad.

Do the work. Feel the difference. Then decide.

ENTERTAIN NO OTHER OPTION

You have a lot of options. Every day you make countless decisions. You can convince yourself of anything. You can talk yourself into or out of doing the work to create change in any and every moment.

You can eat the chips or not. You can accept excuses today or not. You can get in a workout or not. You can work hard or you can ease off. You can sleep in or get up early. You can snap at your loved ones or you can be patient, warm, and kind.

There are options that move you *toward* your goals and options that don't.

There's the path of progress and the path away from progress.

There will always be a reason to do less than your best.

I want to challenge you, even just for today, to entertain no option other than progress. It's the *only* option today.

I'm not suggesting you can't *ever* make a choice that doesn't create progress and momentum, but don't give yourself outs and excuses **today**.

Just start there. Don't let the idea of "weeks" intimidate you. Remember, that's a choice. There's nothing for you to focus on except the day you're in.

I had to use this strategy every day while I was writing this book. I kept trying to talk myself out of writing. I can't. It's too hard. I'm lost. I'm stuck. I'll try again tomorrow.

There's something else I'll work on today. Now's not the time. I'll put it off another year. I'm not ready. Every single day, the idea of writing a book felt daunting.

Without exception, I used this short mantra: entertain no other option.

If I was open to the idea of talking myself out of the work, I always would. I had to remove the option completely, just for the day I was in.

"Later," "tomorrow," and "next week" weren't going to cut it. Not on this day, the day I was in.

No doubt, no delay, no tomorrow—just today.

End the debate. Refuse the delay. Today you work. Today you create progress. Today you choose your goal.

One of the reasons change feels so hard and seems to take so long is because we debate it anew every day. Sometimes we debate it multiple times a day!

Change doesn't feel daunting because you're trying so hard. Change feels daunting because you're not trying hard enough!

Stop giving up so quickly and so often.

I've certainly lived this way. I'd decide that I was going to get healthy and lose weight, but the next morning, I'd be debating Chick-fil-A. A few hours later, I'd be justifying a little bit of ice cream.

It's exhausting! It takes an absurd amount of time and *guarantees* inconsistency.

Not today. Not this time. Not anymore.

It is not an easier way to live. Putting it off doesn't make the journey easier. It makes it infinitely more difficult.

Make up your mind. Pursue progress. Entertain no other option.

Give yourself the experience of maximum effort. You can always go back to the way things have been.

CREATE CHANGE CHALLENGE

Go for it. Take off the emergency brake and put forth your best effort. Stop talking yourself out of the work and instead show yourself what it feels like to work hard, raise your standards, and be the best version of yourself. Commit to this way of living for at least fourteen days. Bonus points for those of you who know you're worth an experience of twenty-one days or more! Take one single day at a time. You always have one excellent day in you!

Pay close attention to what feels hard, but don't submit to it. Remember, you can always go back to the way things were or make changes after this challenge is over, but you need to create this contrast in order to make an informed decision about what feels best.

All the things you crave will be waiting for you after these fourteen days.

Raise your standards and do the work. You deserve this experience. Don't quit. It's time to bring your maximum effort!

As You Go Forward

"You know what the issue is with this world? Everyone wants some magical solution to their problem yet everyone refuses to believe in magic."

—LEWIS CARROLL

I have good news. **You** are the magic. You are the **only** magic you'll ever need.

You have everything you'll ever need, and more, right inside of you, right now.

I smiled when I found this quote because it reflects something I've been saying to my clients since the very beginning of Primal Potential. I get emails every day that say something along the lines of, "Thank you so much! I've transformed my life and it's because of you!"

Nope. It's *not* because of me. It's entirely because of you. You created the change. Just you. *You* are the magic.

Whatever change you want to create next, you have the power to create. You already have everything you need.

Sure, others may inspire and inform you. You can certainly *learn* from great people and have helpful coaches. But change doesn't come from inspiration or information. Change comes from action and only *you* can take those steps and make those choices. Change is purely a result of the **choices** you make and the actions you take when you're on your own. *You* are the only one who can create the change. That means *you* are the magic.

It will work. You can create change. It is possible as soon as you stop giving your energy, thoughts, and attention to all the reasons it won't.

Instead of arguing for what's in the way or what's hard, commit to relentlessly redirect your attention to what you are able and willing to do today to create the change you crave.

You don't need to take notes; you need to take action.

Every choice is a chance. Transformation is now.

Reset Reminders

We all struggle. There is nothing wrong with you. Motivation *naturally* ebbs and flows. Priorities shift. You will get distracted. Welcome to the human experience. This is normal.

Your ability to create change isn't related to whether or not you struggle. You will struggle. **Your ability to create change hinges on how you *respond* to your struggles.**

I've created these reset reminders as simple redirects for you to turn to when you feel stuck, frustrated, powerless, or overwhelmed. You are not stuck. You are not powerless. Feeling overwhelmed and frustrated results from your perspective, not your circumstances. You can change your perspective right now.

These reset reminders are simple because they do not

need to be complex. Shifting momentum and attention is not complicated.

You are always able to move immediately from struggle to success.

WHAT ARE YOU CHASING?

What do you want most? Act like it.

LET IT GO

Stop clinging to what is behind you. It's over. If you are giving energy to the problem, you're keeping it from the solution. You are a problem *solver*—a creative, energetic problem solver. Take action. What is the next best choice you can make? Do it now, then do it again.

ONE GOOD CHOICE

You have one good choice in you. Excellence is the next five minutes. It doesn't matter how much there is to do or how far you have to go. Be where your feet are. Win the moment you're in.

YOU'RE NOT A VICTIM

You are not a victim of your circumstances. End the

drama. I'm sure you're busy and life feels hard. Do you want to be a victim or a victor? There is no circumstance that removes your power to make a great choice. There is a difference between making yourself better and simply making yourself *feel* better. You are just a few great choices away from feeling in control. In this moment, **be** better. Think differently. Transformation is now!

THERE'S PLENTY YOU CAN DO

Time is up. Give no more attention to what you can't do. There will be no more complaining or explaining about your obstacles or limitations. There's plenty you *can* do. If you were hiking a mountain, would it help you to focus on how steep it is, how many rocks are in the ground, or the falling rain? It would not. What *can* you do? Do that.

OVERCOME TEMPTATION

Refuse to lose sight of what you really want. You will face temptation. Are you willing to trade this temptation for that goal? Is it worth it? Is your dream for sale? Really? Do you think it will be worth it *this* time? Stop holding yourself back. You are so close to the amazing life you desire, but you cannot get there if you keep saying no to the goal and yes to the temptation.

IT IS POSSIBLE

It is possible. You are capable. The goal you're seeking is closer than you think, but it requires that you dig in and do the work. It is worth it! Develop that competitive stamina! *You* are worth it! This choice on this day is an opportunity to advance. Say yes to your better life. Buckle down and earn it.

Create your own reset reminder. What do you need to hear in the hard moments? Write a short message that brings you back to power and progress and share it with me by tagging @elizabethbenton on Instagram!

Two-Hundred-Plus Questions That Can Change Your Life

Adopting a better set of questions will create a better life. The power of these questions comes from asking them regularly, answering them honestly, and taking action on your answers.

These questions aren't here for you to sit and answer. Use them daily to help you create change, overcome temptation, and become a better version of yourself. You'll find that some questions motivate and inspire you more than others. Use those first.

Over time, you might find that they don't create the impact on your choices that they once did. At that point, start asking different questions.

As you grow and change, the questions that impact you will change, too.

If you feel stuck on any of the questions or answers, here are some universal follow-ups that can move you from thought into action.

Now what?

What will I do about this today?

What other options do I have?

How can I change this?

Is it working?

Here's to creating your very best life and chasing your highest potential, one question at a time!

....

What are you chasing?

What's *worth* chasing?

What do you need to let go of?

What's in the way?

Who do you want to become?

What can you do about it today?

Why do you stay in prison when the door is so wide open?

What can you release that is no longer serving you?

What can you release that is causing unnecessary tension?

What's the difference, in your own life, between learning and changing?

What are you rushing?

Why?

Is that your best approach?

What other options are there?

How can you practice being militantly on your own side?

In your own life, what's the difference between evolution and revolution?

How is solving your problem different from responding to it?

What's the difference, in your own life, between doing things right and doing the right things?

What do you want most?

What change do you want to create?

What are you afraid to let go of?

Why?

How might you benefit from letting go?

In what ways are you cutting corners?

Are you cheating yourself?

In what ways do you travel along the hard road?

How can you make it easier?

In what ways have you let yourself down?

What familiar and convenient lies do you tell yourself?

What are you in the habit of putting off?

What is your go-to approach that doesn't work?

In what ways do you let emotions cloud your decisions?

What does it look like for you to value consistency over intensity?

What can you do today that you've been putting off?

In what ways would you benefit from improving your mindset?

What can you do today to improve your mindset?

What does it look like to make your decisions based on principle instead of emotion?

How can you practice?

What are some of your white-knuckle approaches?

Do they work?

What might work better?

How can you work with yourself instead of against yourself?

Are you giving yourself credit for trying?

Is it working?

Are you where you want to be?

Are you moving in the right direction?

Is your pace acceptable to you?

In what ways do you justify your lack of progress?

How do you differentiate between effort and progress?

What do you know you need to do?

Where are there gaps between what you know and what you do?

How will you close those gaps this week?

Are you attracted to the accumulation of information?

How can you use some of that time and energy on action?

In what ways are you contributing to the problem?

How can you be a vibrant change agent in your life today?

In what ways are you *practicing* the problem?

How can you practice the solution?

How will you take control?

How can you create excellence in the next five minutes?

What is the next great choice you will make?

How will you win the moment you're in?

What if, just for one day, you seized every single moment and every single choice as a chance to move in the direction of your goals?

Are you willing to try that?

Will you do it today?

Why wait?

What are three opportunities you can seize today to create transformation?

How will you remind yourself to choose transformation every day this week?

Where do you have opportunities for improvement in your actions, thoughts, or reactions today?

What will you implement today to intentionally redirect your thoughts and attention to the present moment?

Are you practicing the best version of yourself?

In what ways are you hesitating?

What can you do today that will make tomorrow easier?

What is slowing you down?

What is in the way of your progress?

What do you need to remove from your life?

Are you willing to let go of your past?

Are your intentions and your attention aligned?

Is what you want possible?

Do you believe more in your past or your potential?

Are you acting like it?

Will you cling to fear or chase your growth?

What beliefs do you need to cut yourself off from?

What are some behaviors, thoughts, patterns, or habits that don't reflect the best version of you?

In what ways do you fuel them with your thoughts, attention, or choices?

How might you make today different?

What limitations do you argue for?

How?

What else is true?

What change can you make this week to make other parts of your life flow more easily?

What stories are slowing you down?

What problems or fears do you believe in?

What else is possible?

What do you believe about areas where you struggle?

What do you believe about areas where you're thriving?

What's the difference?

What do you believe about your potential for change?

What do you believe about who you are and how you act, as it relates to your goal?

What stories are you holding on to that you can choose to leave in the past?

How can you change your story to improve your results?

What thoughts do you need to stop fueling with your attention and emotion?

What behaviors predict or influence your goal?

What behaviors predict or influence your failure?

What thoughts drive your excuses?

What thoughts drive your success?

How can you focus today on changing your thoughts about your challenges or goals?

How can you pay more attention to your thoughts?

How can you practice thinking differently?

What were you thinking when you made that choice?

In what ways do you make things worse?

Where are you telling incomplete truths to justify all-or-nothing behaviors?

What is the whole truth you are avoiding?

What do you know about what doesn't work for you?

How can you avoid approaches that don't work for you today?

What's a middle ground between your excuse and your intention?

What are some neutral redirects you can practice?

What are some positive redirects you can practice?

What are some empowering redirects you can practice?

Which of your thoughts do you need to practice redirecting?

What types of thoughts aren't relevant?

In what ways are you wasting time or energy?

What drains your energy or drive?

What will you do about it?

How do you talk yourself into all-or-nothing approaches?

What alternative perspectives can you practice?

What happens when you choose an all-or-nothing approach?

Why do you want to achieve your goal?

What will it change?

What is it that you'll have, be, experience, or feel when you reach your goal that you don't have now?

What do you want to feel that you don't feel now?

What do you want more of in your life?

What do you want less of?

What contributes to your happiness?

What contributes to your unhappiness?

What makes you feel calm?

What arouses your stress or anxiety?

What are your internal goals?

What are your external targets?

What can you do to pursue that internal target separately, instead of assuming it will come along with the achievement of the external goal?

When you get to the end of your life, how would you have to have lived to consider it a great success?

How do you define a happy life?

What are the gaps between that happy life you've defined and the life you're living now?

What can you do today to begin to bridge the gap?

What are three ways you can move closer to a happier life?

What choices erode your happiness, confidence, or peace of mind?

In your own life, what's the difference between relational work and problem-solving work?

How do you differentiate between sensing and solving?

What are some interesting options you have?

In what ways are you settling?

What will you do the next time you feel stuck?

To what problems are you not applying creative, energetic solutions?

On what problems can you practice?

What would it look like?

If someone else were in charge of solving the problems in your life, what would you want them to do?

How can you be more creative and energetic in the way you solve problems in your life?

In which of the phases of the problem are you wasting energy: sensing, seeking, settling, or solving?

Where do you need to spend more time?

Do you have a dream or a goal?

What's the difference?

How can you decrease the amount of time between a bad choice and the next good one?

What ways of thinking do you need to challenge or reframe?

Are you fooling yourself?

Are you lying to yourself?

What closed cases do you reopen?

Which of your answers isn't the truth?

What's the difference between being right and getting it right?

What is the truth that moves you forward?

How can you recognize when you're under the influence of emotion?

What assumptions are you making?

Are you creating drama?

If you showed up in this moment as the person you want to be, what choice would you make?

What emotions are clouding your decision-making right now?

What is the difference between what happened and what you're telling yourself happened?

What is the difference between what happened and how you feel about what happened?

What meaning have you attached to the situation?

What is the full version of the truth?

What have you not considered?

What else is true?

What choice will make you proud?

What is the simplest solution?

Are you focused?

Where are you adding unnecessary complexity?

How can you simplify things?

What small wins can you create today?

What do you dismiss as too small to matter?

What baby steps are you able to take today?

What simple daily disciplines do you need to establish as habits?

How will you invest in yourself today?

What simple decision-making criteria can you employ?

In one sentence, what is the problem?

Are you looking for attention or are you looking for a solution?

Are you in the stands or in the game?

What's the difference?

What are you afraid to miss out on?

What does "more" add to your life?

If you say yes, what are you saying no to?

What will happen if this behavior continues?

Are you willing to choose short-term sacrifice for long-term reward?

How will you recognize the lie of FOMO the next time it comes up?

What is the reputation you have with yourself?

What is the reputation you want to have?

What will you do today to improve that reputation?

What is the behavior you wish you'd effortlessly demonstrate in this situation?

What does it mean to you to be whole and undivided?

Will you be someone who does what is right or someone who does what is easy?

What do you need to ignore?

What will you do today to build butt power?

Do you know what sustained maximum effort feels like?

Are you willing to create that experience for yourself?

What do you have to lose?

Do you know how amazing you can feel?

What will you do to make today amazing?

Acknowledgments

Mom, my first and best teacher: Thank you for your bravery and openness. Sharing our story has healed us and thousands of others. Thank you for loving me exactly as you did. I wouldn't change a thing.

Grandpa: You are the source of my strength. Thank you for teaching me to be relentless.

Debi: Your steadfast support is my foundation. God knew what He was doing when He made us sisters.

Kathi: You were the first to lovingly teach me that I could reinvent myself at any age, in any moment. I love you and your unwavering example of creativity and persistence.

Andrew: My best friend and sounding board. Thanks for

helping me become a better version of myself and for your patience and love along the way.

Chris: Without your endless encouragement, I wouldn't have finished this book. I'm glad I didn't count the number of times you lectured me to get back to writing, but it made a difference. Thanks for believing in me and holding me to a high standard.

Dave Ramsey and team: Thank you for teaching me to create financial peace—it was the first step toward personal freedom and an incredible life.

To my family, friends, and clients: It takes a village. Thank you for your support and for being a part of my journey. This is only the beginning.

About the Author

With a degree in human nutrition from University of North Carolina, Greensboro, ELIZABETH BENTON became a nutritionist to help others find relief from obesity. Struggling with obesity herself, she was lost in a world of depression, which led to pain, debt, and marriage problems—all while educating thousands of people about nutrition and weight management in her management role with a large dietary supplement company. Finally, she realized that more education wasn't the answer. She had to take the leap and save herself. She couldn't just learn about change, she had to implement it.

At just thirty-five years old, Elizabeth Benton is the founder and creator of Primal Potential, an online education company that helps people create transformations through podcasts, courses, coaching programs, and live events. Her podcasts focus 70 percent on mindset and 30 percent on hormones and nutrition, recognizing that people don't lack knowledge, but the tools to consistently implement that knowledge.

Made in the USA
Middletown, DE
16 September 2022

10627848R00224